Praise for *Health Shift*

"Dr. Alice Burron has written a complete blueprint for anyone who wishes to understand how to deal with health challenges and achieve optimal health. I have been in the health and fitness field for over thirty years and still felt like my entire understanding of the field was given a huge 'upgrade' by reading this book!"

—DR. MARK BRITTINGHAM, PHD, president, BSDI

"Dr. Burron has adeptly synthesized the literature on health behavior change, self-efficacy, and identity, assembled the most relevant elements, and then taken them a step further to make them understandable and doable, with added food for thought that many likely do not consider. I love the Surreptitious Seven Tendencies! They fill a gap in awareness of the influences on decision-making and action. Each point is fuel for some serious contemplation and introspection."

—LISA ELSINGER, PHD

"It's time to rethink how we approach health and healthcare. The two are often intertwined, but our personal health choices ultimately shape our well-being. *Health Shift* empowers us to take a more holistic approach, expanding our understanding of both traditional and alternative options. By shifting our mindset, we can move from a 'sick care' system to true health care—one that prioritizes prevention, education, and lasting well-being."

—KIM FARMER, corporate wellness specialist, Mile High Fitness and Wellness

"Dr. Burron's *Health Shift* invites us to expand our perspective, seamlessly integrating both conventional and complementary approaches to well-being. For too long, healthcare has centered on treating illness rather than championing the power of prevention. Through her eloquent words, she masterfully weaves a message of transformation—one that urges us to shift our mindset and take an active role in our own health. Rather than dwelling on what needs to be 'fixed,' *Health Shift* empowers individuals to reclaim their well-being, instilling the confidence to advocate for a healthier, more vibrant life."

—DR. ERIN NITSCHKE, EdD, American Council on Exercise (ACE) Scientific Advisory Committee member

HEALTH SHIFT

YOUR PERSONALIZED
GUIDE TO MAKING STRATEGIC
HEALTH DECISIONS

DR. ALICE BURRON

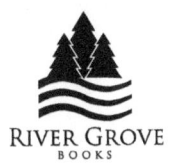

RIVER GROVE
BOOKS

This book is intended as a reference resource and should not be considered a medical manual or a substitute for professional medical advice. The information provided is designed to assist readers in making informed decisions about their health. It is not intended to replace any treatment prescribed by a licensed healthcare professional. If you suspect a medical condition, please consult a qualified healthcare provider.

The author assumes no responsibility or liability for any loss, damage, or injury caused or alleged to be caused directly or indirectly by the use or application of the information contained in this book.

Additionally, names and identifying details of individuals mentioned in this work have been altered to protect their privacy.

Published by River Grove Books
Austin, TX
www.rivergrovebooks.com

Copyright © 2025 2BFIT, LLC

All rights reserved.

Thank you for purchasing an authorized edition of this book and for complying with copyright law. No part of this book may be reproduced, stored in a retrieval system, or transmitted by any means, electronic, mechanical, photocopying, recording, or otherwise, without written permission from the copyright holder.

Distributed by River Grove Books

Design and composition by Greenleaf Book Group and Kim Lance
Cover design by Greenleaf Book Group and Kim Lance
Health Hero character and map illustrations are by Laura Dreyer.
Used with permission.

Publisher's Cataloging-in-Publication data is available.

Print ISBN: 978-1-63299-984-9

eBook ISBN: 978-1-63299-985-6

First Edition

Contents

INTRODUCTION
Taking Control of Your Health Destiny ... 1

PART I
Conquering the Forces Working Against You ... 9
1. Turning Complacency into Curiosity. 11
2. Recognizing Thinking That May Be Holding You Back. 23
3. Swimming Upstream in the Culture Current 37
4. Navigating a Complex Information Landscape 51

PART II
Developing Your Health Hero Superpowers ... 69
5. Defining Your Compass: A Health Philosophy for Balance and Harmony. 71
6. Taking Control of Your Decisions 85
7. From Personality to Reality: Using Decision-Making Tools . . . 103
8. Developing Confidence Through Belief and Attitude. 119
9. Naming the Unnamed: Being Able to Articulate Your Emotions 137

PART III
Making Healing Happen: Your Action Plan ... 149
10. How Is Your Health . . . Really? 151
11. CREECS: Defining Your Health Approach (The Six Questions Everyone Should Answer Before Making Any Health Decision) 167

12	Lifestyle Interventions, Part 1: The Core 4	181
13	Lifestyle Interventions, Part 2: Expanding Your Arsenal of Health Tools	199
14	Getting the Most from Conventional Medicine	213
15	Unlocking the Power of Complementary Healing	227
16	Creating a Healing Action Plan Just for You	241

CONCLUSION
Envisioning the Journey to a HEALTHIER You   **263**

Acknowledgments *269*
Notes *271*
About the Author *281*

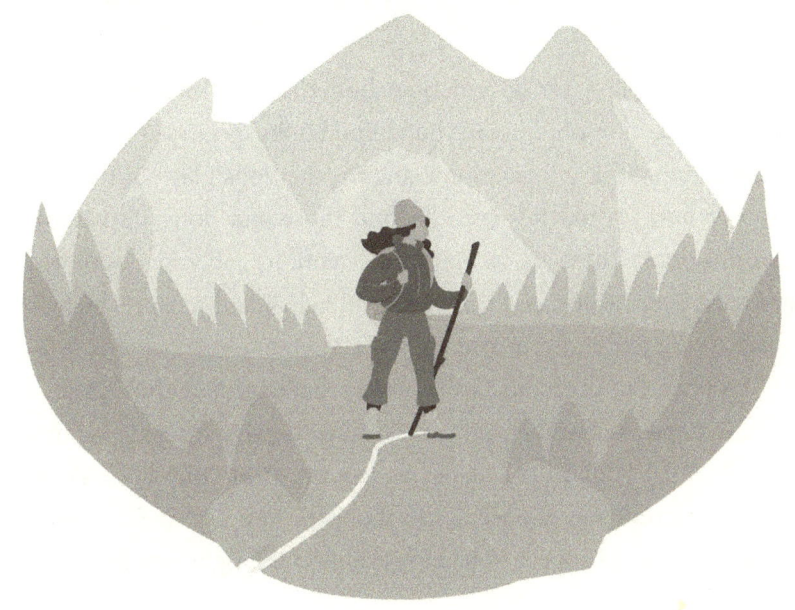

INTRODUCTION

Taking Control of Your Health Destiny

This book is about healing faster. And it's also about hope. I'm profoundly hopeful about your ability to heal faster than you ever have before. Everyone is dealing with one health issue or another or trying to stay healthy in an unsupportive environment for optimal health. Finding an easy way to get better and stay healthy has never been more elusive.

Whether you're dealing with a condition like lupus, chronic fatigue syndrome, or diabetes; or grappling with persistent symptoms like headaches, anxiety, and heart palpitations; or dealing with something like high blood pressure, I want you to know that you have more power to improve and overcome whatever is impeding your best health. I'll help you get to the root of the issue and connect you to the best possible solution for you.

If you're looking for information about the exact intervention to heal your health condition, I invite you to find books specific to your particular condition. Seek information using the methods I lay out for you and discover new approaches even beyond those, but don't start until you read this book. There are so many interventions and varieties of ways to approach your health, and this book will help you discover which one is worth trying and right for you.

The power to overcome your health challenge is within reach—and there is hope. Remember, no one else can do this for you; it's in your court to turn your health concern around. And your hope is not in the intervention you choose, it's in the tactic you use. We'll explore the unlimited ways to approach healing and find the right way for you. It all starts with a shift in thinking.

Using my background in health sciences and health improvement, combined with practical strategies that simplify health choices, I developed an innovative approach to help people cut through the confusion of what to do next and find what truly works for them. I've coached numerous individuals to overcome overwhelm and feel empowered, confident, and in control of their next steps, so they can move forward knowing they're doing their best to overcome their health concerns.

Take Sarah and Mark, for example—two of my clients who each battled long-term health issues. Sarah had lived with chronic pain for years, and Mark was weighed down by chronic depression. Both had accepted their conditions as part of life, convinced that true healing was beyond their reach. But something incredible happened when they began questioning those beliefs. Sarah realized that she had lost hope of ever feeling pain-free, and Mark had resigned himself to the idea that depression was just part of his identity. The moment they opened their minds to the possibility of change, their healing journeys began.

By embracing curiosity and challenging the limits they'd placed on their own potential, Sarah and Mark started to think with hope and belief. This mental shift sparked something profound. As their brains rewired, they began to see new opportunities for healing—approaches and methods they had never considered before. And as they explored these new possibilities, something even more remarkable happened: their bodies responded. Gradually, they felt the effects of their changing mindset influencing their physical health. Today, both Sarah and Mark are fully restored and living healthy, vibrant lives.

It wasn't some miracle or magical cure that turned their health around. It was the simple yet powerful willingness to open their minds to new ideas and approaches. They rewrote their health stories, and so can you.

This book is all about helping you cultivate the mindset and philosophy behind smart health decisions. You will soon be able to navigate the maze of misinformation, cultural pressures, and be prepared for the maddeningly complex healthcare system, should you need it. After reading this book, you will become a **Health Hero**. The images used in this guide are of Health Hero Girl, or Hero Girl. Hero Girl represents you—curious, smart, strategic, and able to overcome any health obstacle. Use her to inspire you as you move forward on this amazing journey of healing and health discovery.

The Secret Weapons of a Health Hero

The statistics are alarming: six in ten adults in the U.S. suffer from chronic diseases, and more than half of them have multiple conditions.[1] Instead of accepting this as the norm, we need to rekindle our curiosity, which drives us to ask, "Is there a better way?"

I've been seeking the answer to that question for several decades, through a career that spans working in the healthcare system, health insurance industry, as a personal trainer, and holding a doctoral degree in healthcare education and leadership. This book is the result of that work, and I offer it as a novel way for you to seek the answers you deserve by asking the right questions.

The approach I've developed is embodied in the concept of **Health Heroes**—individuals who are taking back control and actively shaping their own health journey. Health Heroes don't rush to Dr. Google to find the answers to all their health questions. Instead, they develop their power to control their health by . . .

- believing in their **body's ability to heal** (and knowing how to use their intuition, self-awareness, logic, and emotional intelligence to catalyze the healing process);
- being **curious** and **humble** and keeping their minds open to new pathways to better health;
- preferring **knowledge** over ignorance, **reality** over assumptions;
- staying alert to the ways in which our society and media may be **biasing their beliefs;**
- understanding how their **personality** and **attitudes** may be helping or hindering their ability to make good decisions about their health; and
- understanding that an effective healthcare approach must be **unique to them**: approaches or treatments that work for another person may not work for them.

I'm willing to bet many of the items on this list are topics you haven't come across in other books or articles about health. That's a big part of what makes this book stand out from the rest. Many health books tend to focus on just one aspect of managing well-being, but they often overlook the importance of a holistic approach to making intentional, informed health decisions—no matter what condition you're dealing with. This book is different. It guides you through a comprehensive process, empowering you to make the best choices for your unique situation.

In the later chapters, we explore each of the Health Hero attributes in more depth. But before we dive in, I'd like to introduce you to a special feature of the book: the Health Hero perspectives. These key insights, woven throughout the chapters, highlight the essential mindset of a Health Hero and will guide you on your journey to better health. Just look for the Health Hero image and accompanying text.

What I want to emphasize is that becoming a Health Hero is more than just a title—it represents a complete shift in mindset. It's about moving away from the conventional focus on "what" to try to fix a health issue and instead dives into the deeper, more powerful "why."

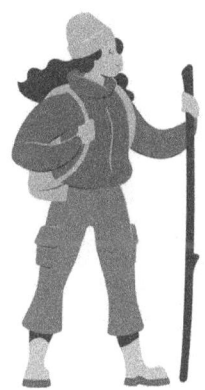

By reading this book, you'll actively engage in practicing curiosity, challenging assumptions, and exploring new perspectives on your health.

In our fast-paced world, it's easy to get caught up in the "what"—the treatments, diets, medications, or beauty procedures we think will fix the problem. We're constantly bombarded with the next big health intervention, whether it's a trendy diet, a new weight loss drug, or an unnecessary procedure. Choosing a convenient health fix is understandable because when a health concern arises, the natural reaction is to want to fix it immediately. But these seemingly perfectly timed interventions fail to address the root of the issue.

Health Heroes understand that addressing a health concern starts with a deeper exploration—before deciding *what* to do, they first seek to uncover *why* the issue arose in the first place. It's this foundational "why" that gives meaning and clarity to the "what." Without understanding the root cause, any action taken is merely a guess. But when the "why" is illuminated, the "what" becomes a natural, logical response, ensuring that the chosen path is not only effective but truly aligned with what the body and mind need. True healing happens when we reverse the typical approach—let the "why" lead, and the "what" will follow with purpose and precision.

Health Heroes Rescue Themselves

Another unique feature of this book is that it is NOT about a one-size-fits-all solution; it's a manual for navigating the complex and often confusing world of health. And it's for everyone—whether you're facing a health crisis, just trying to stay well, or working with others as a healthcare professional in the field.

The truth is that no one is coming to rescue us from our health issues—we must be our own Health Heroes or have one in our corner. This book is your guide, your manual, to help you live empowered, curious, and healthier than ever before. It's time to embrace our health fully, not just manage it. Together, we can transform how we approach healing, not by waiting for a broken healthcare system to fix itself, but by taking charge of our own health journey. We need a movement of Health Heroes taking over the nation to make our country healthy again.

To help you become a Health Hero, this book is divided into three transformative parts that will not only reveal the forces working against you but also arm you with the tools you need to conquer them and make the best health decisions possible:

Part I: Conquering the Forces Working Against You—Prepare to uncover the hidden dangers that are quietly but powerfully impacting your health and decision-making. Most of us go through life unaware of these threats, but it's time to see the health landscape for what it truly is—riddled with challenges that can undermine your well-being. In chapters 1 to 4, I take you on a journey to reveal the most pervasive external factors standing in the way of your health success. Once you understand these forces, you'll be ready to strategize and overcome them, becoming stronger and more prepared to protect your health.

Part II: Developing Your Health Hero Superpowers—Every great hero has to tap into their unique strengths, and you are no different. But before you can unlock your superpowers, you need to recognize your internal limits and turn them into strengths. In this section, you discover how self-awareness, personality, attitudes, and emotions play a huge role in your health decisions. Chapters 5 to 9 are designed to help you develop the essential qualities of a Health Hero, enabling you to understand yourself more deeply and harness the power of your thoughts to heal. You'll learn how to transform your mindset, and I'll show you how this shift can drive your healing journey.

Part III: Making Healing Happen (Your Action Plan)—Now comes the exciting part! In chapters 10 to 16, you'll pull everything together and create a personalized Healing Action Plan that's aligned with your beliefs, customized to your body's needs, and inclusive of a range of treatments—whether lifestyle, complementary, or traditional medical interventions. Healing is not a one-size-fits-all process, and I guide you through discovering the options that work best for you. You'll develop a unique health approach where your plan is entirely your own, built around your values, preferences, and goals. No one else will have the same plan, because no one else is you.

It's time to rethink how you manage your health so you can heal faster, and I'm ready to show you how to empower yourself to be healthier than you ever have been before. Are you ready? Let's get started on your new journey to becoming a Health Hero!

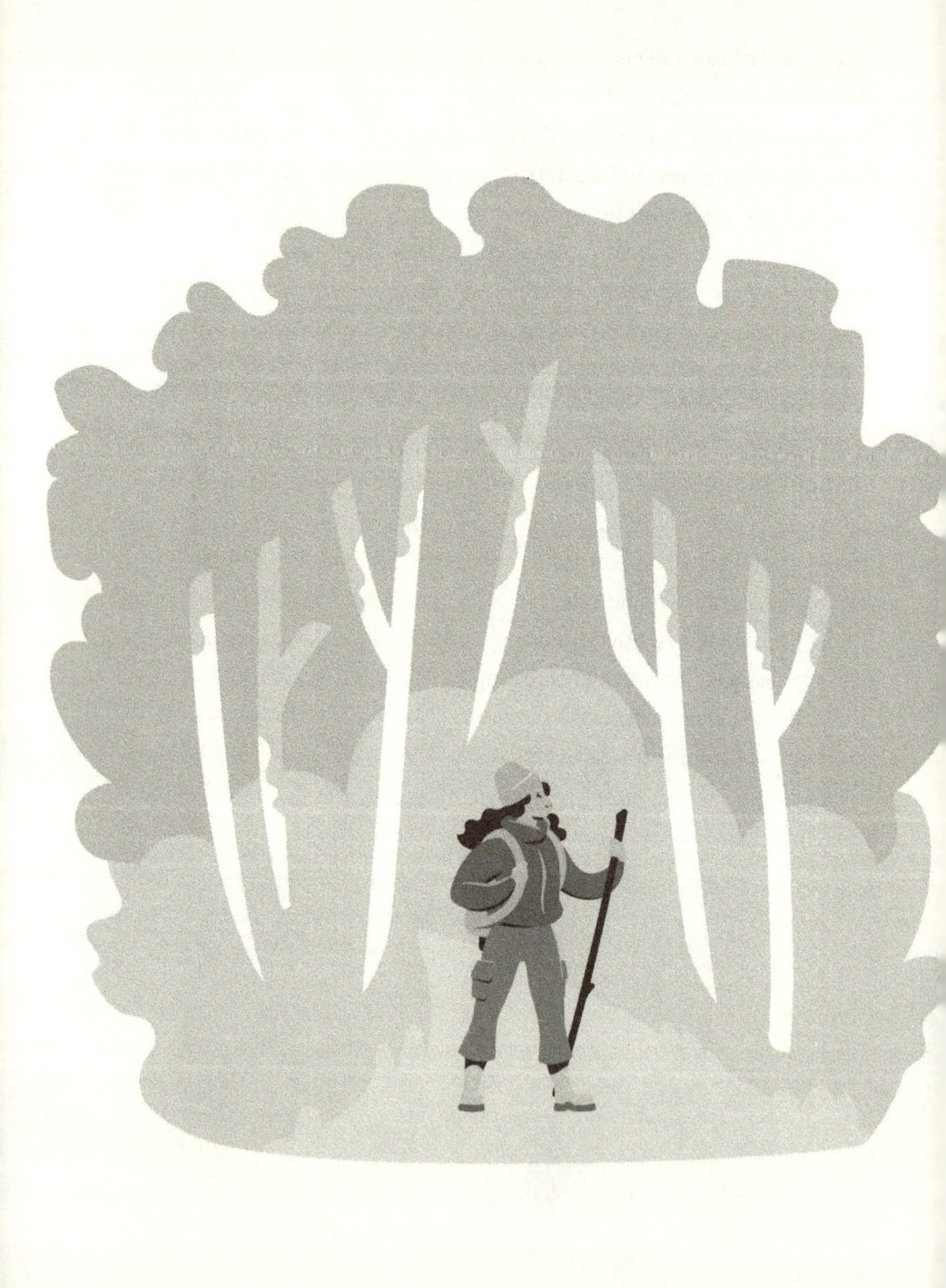

Part I

Conquering the Forces Working Against You

In our everyday lives, it's all too easy to feel more like a victim than a superhero when it comes to our health. The truth is, we're up against powerful forces that often seem determined to undermine our well-being. The healthcare system can feel like a maze, with barriers at every turn. In fact, nearly 65 percent of Americans feel overwhelmed by the complexity of the healthcare system, often leading to delayed or avoided care.[1] Meanwhile, healthy foods are not only harder to find but can be up to 60 percent more expensive than processed alternatives, making it all too tempting to reach for the junk food.[2] And let's not forget the constant bombardment of advertising—whether it's the latest diet, supplement, or miracle cure—that promises to solve all our problems, but rarely delivers.

These forces are not just inconveniences; they're roadblocks that can prevent us from making informed, healthy choices. If we don't recognize and actively fight against them, we risk losing control of our health altogether. But here's the good news: you are the owner of your health destiny. It's time to take back the reins, and that journey begins by understanding the forces working against you.

By reading this book, you'll gain the knowledge and tools to break free from these challenges. No longer will you be a victim of the forces conspiring against your health. Instead, you'll be empowered to make informed decisions that truly benefit your well-being.

In part I of this book, we explore how to turn complacency into curiosity, break free from unhelpful thinking patterns, swim against the current of a culture that often prioritizes profit over health, and navigate the overwhelming landscape of information that can either mislead or empower you.

This isn't just about making better choices—it's about reclaiming your power and becoming the hero of your own health story. By the time you finish part I, you'll be equipped to face these forces head-on, ensuring they no longer have the power to dictate your health journey.

Here's how we'll do it:

- Turn complacency into curiosity (chapter 1)
- Recognize thinking patterns that may be holding you back (chapter 2)
- Learn how to swim upstream in the culture current (chapter 3)
- Know how to navigate a complex information landscape (chapter 4)

The journey to better health starts with understanding the battlefield. Let's begin.

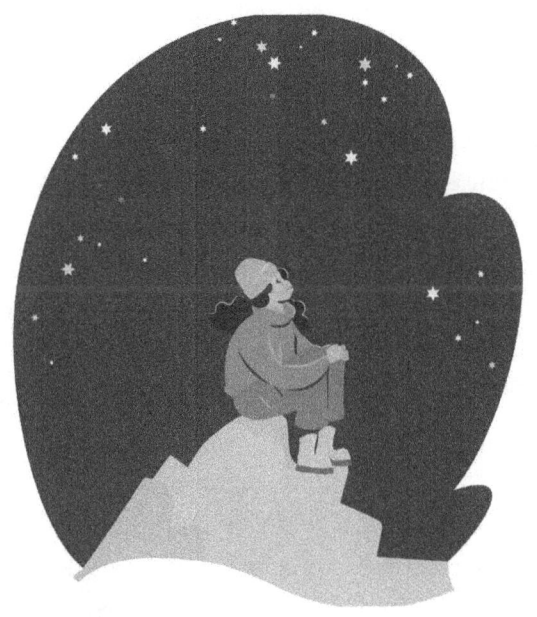

CHAPTER 1

Turning Complacency into Curiosity

Many people come to me feeling uncertain about issues like high cholesterol or blood pressure. Their doctors have prescribed medication, but they're hesitant—unsure if they should take it or if there might be another way. Often, they have an unspoken philosophy: they'd rather try something else before relying on medication. I applaud that mindset because it reflects a thoughtful approach to health, and I'm always eager to guide them through alternative interventions.

More often than not, with a little guidance and curiosity, my clients are able to lower their numbers into a healthy range within a few months—without medication. Their openness to explore different intervention modalities—like research-backed supplements, nutrition adjustments, physical activity, and stress management—makes all the difference. It's this curiosity, this willingness to look beyond the first option, that opens the door to new ways of healing.

But even for those who ultimately choose to take medication, there's a sense of peace in knowing they explored all their options. They didn't settle for a quick fix—they made an informed decision, and that alone gives them confidence and contentment. And that's what I want for you. I want you to understand just how much untapped potential you have to overcome health concerns. No matter what ailments you face, you have the capability to approach your health with newfound confidence.

Unfortunately, most people don't approach health this way. We live in a quick-fix culture that prioritizes treating conditions after they appear rather than focusing on prevention and continuous healing. While this treatment mentality might work for some health issues, it falls short for many. If we continue to handle our health in the same reactive way, we'll remain trapped in a cycle of treating, not healing—leading to a society that's perpetually sick rather than typically healthy.

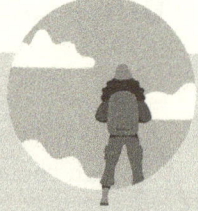

Q&A WITH ALICE: QUICK FIXES

Many people tell me that they are drawn to quick fixes, whether it be a new supplement, diet, or medication. "I know they're not long-term solutions," people tell me, "but I can't help myself. What should I do to not be persuaded to try quick-fix approaches?"

> It's understandable to feel the allure of quick fixes, especially when we all want fast results. However, true health requires consistent effort and sustainable habits. Quick fixes might offer temporary benefits, but they often don't address the root of the problem. Try shifting your focus to long-term well-being rather than instant results. Ask yourself: "Is this a Band-Aid, or is it a real solution?" Gradually, you'll find that the deeper, more lasting approaches bring the real changes you're seeking. Start small, celebrate incremental progress, and remind yourself that true health is a journey, not a sprint.

Over the years, I've come to believe that learning how to make better health decisions is one of the biggest challenges we face—not just as individuals, but as a nation. This book is about how we can become powerful Health Heroes, capable of taking control of our well-being.

So, let's begin this journey by exploring why it's so difficult for us to make good health decisions. And let's uncover why humility and curiosity may just be the most powerful superpower you can wield to counteract the self-defeating tendencies that hold you back from being at your best health.

The Surreptitious Seven Tendencies: Why It's Hard to Make Good Health Decisions

I bet that you, like most of us, have a vision of yourself in the future that assumes you are healthy. You're walking down a beach, hand in hand with your partner, or you're getting together with friends eating at a nice dining spot. Maybe you're hiking a trail high in the mountaintops. But the reality is, most of us have tendencies that move us away from that healthy vision we see ourselves in. We don't realize that our blood sugar is in the danger zone, where diabetes may result. There will be no extreme adventurous hike if that happens. The vision at the restaurant will change drastically as we peruse through the menu and see that many items will not be ones we can enjoy, because of our diabetes. This is the future we are advancing to, but we still don't see ourselves that way. It's time to be honest with our situation and what we envision for ourselves. Otherwise, we are hindering our own progress and outcomes—our best future is at stake. So, the first step is to discover ourselves and our tendencies that are getting in the way of our best future self. The most dangerous of these are what I call the Surreptitious Seven Tendencies.

The first, and perhaps the most prevalent, tendency of the seven is our natural inclination **to react, and often overreact, to a health scare rather than preventing it in the first place.**[1] I get that life is busy and the demands that are placed on us are overpowering at times. But if you want to unleash the Health Hero within you, you must anticipate the obstacles to your best health. Know when your health is potentially jeopardized. For example, anticipate that your gut won't like when you eat that greasy burger again tonight, or your teeth will pay the price if you don't floss. You may even want to envision yourself in the future and see what your action today will do to that vision—that vision of yourself in the future. What if you don't have any teeth because you didn't floss, as you smile lovingly with several teeth missing at your partner while holding hands walking down the beach? Now think about what you can do today to make your desired vision tomorrow a reality. In this case, I guarantee that flossing will come easier if you think of that toothless smile, trust me.

The second **tendency is ignoring our body's invaluable signals and reactions.**[2] Life's hustle and bustle often leads us to overlook the whispers of our own bodies, those gentle nudges and subtle cues that hint at our well-being. We forge ahead, often disregarding these early warning signs, until our bodies resort to shouting to capture our attention. Do you have tight shoulders at the end of the day, often experience a headache, or maybe you are feeling anxious or depressed? Left unheard, these signals become stronger, until they're forcing your attention. By then, it will take some heavier effort to resolve those issues. It would be much better to listen and address the issues early on.

> ### Listening to Our Bodies
>
> Our bodies often give us early warning signs of underlying issues long before they develop into serious health concerns. Subtle symptoms like fatigue, headaches, digestive changes, or persistent aches are our body's way of signaling that something isn't right. However, these cues are easy to overlook until they reach a tipping point that demands immediate action. As C.S. Lewis wisely observed, "Pain insists on being attended to." Yet, if we intervene early, a gentle approach may be enough to restore our health.
>
> By pausing to reflect on when these symptoms first appeared, we might realize our bodies had been trying to communicate for some time. Addressing these early signals can prevent more serious complications. Sometimes, a week of rest, mindful stress management, or a shift in diet is all it takes to regain balance. On the other hand, waiting until the issue worsens will require more aggressive interventions. Practicing awareness of your body's subtle cues before they become urgent alarms allows you to respond in a way that promotes healing, with the need to treat. Remember, symptoms are your body's way of asking for help. Symptoms exist so you can take steps to heal.

The third tendency involves how you feel about what's happening with your health and **the influence of your feelings on your health**

decisions.[3] Our emotional selves, while a beautiful part of being human, can sometimes lead us astray when it comes to making sound health decisions. We may find ourselves overwhelmed by fear, anxiety, or stress, making choices that don't align with our well-being. Conversely, we might downplay the significance of our emotions, thus unintentionally ignoring the deep impact they can have on our physical health. Our health decisions can also be clouded by irrational thinking patterns influenced by unhelpful biases and other thinking tendencies we've adopted, leading us to make choices that don't align with our best interests. Observe your emotions and how they're impacting your health decisions. We explore how you can become emotionally intelligent and use emotions to help you on the path to healing in later chapters.

The fourth tendency is **a failure to pick out the signal from the noise when it comes to health information.**[4] We're being persuaded every day to try different cures or treatments so we can look our best, be our healthiest, and overcome our specific conditions. It's all too easy to succumb to the temptation to try the quick fix or get overwhelmed with too much information. The result is that we agree to try whatever randomly comes our way. You can see why this is not the best approach for managing your health. Whatever we commit to in the moment will quickly be discarded or we'll pay the price, financially and physically.

The fifth of the Surreptitious Seven is **a failure to recognize alternative options**. We've been socially conditioned to think that we should always seek a doctor's opinion first.[5] I'm not saying that we shouldn't discuss concerns with physicians. I love doctors—they have helped me and my family tremendously. But we should seek a doctor's advice within a framework of understanding how they can and *cannot* help us. Many times, we can control our health and healing if we're open to exploring different avenues for health improvement first, before going to the doctor. We can positively impact our health through varied options, such as nutrition, activity, and complementary therapies—we just need to tap into that vast world of intervention options. In later chapters you'll see some of the options available to you, and it will open the door to a whole new way of approaching your health issues.

The sixth challenge—a tendency that we could easily counter—is **our failure to strategically evaluate our health and health improvement efforts.** A symptom pops up and we counter it with a supplement or an exercise, or a practice, like mindfulness or EFT (emotional freedom techniques) or "tapping," with hopes that it helps us feel better. Yet few of us track our symptom intensity after implementing these techniques to gauge their effectiveness. Typically, our patience runs out after a week or two and we quit before seeing any benefit.

The last of the Surreptitious Seven is one of those most often overlooked. Yet it is imperative for us to overcome this obstacle to be able to approach our health with all engines firing. What is this roadblock to healing? **A lack of health humility.** Health humility is the understanding that we don't have all the answers, that we aren't always the experts in our health, and it opens the gate to approach our health with an open mind, so we expand our options. Without health humility, we risk being blinded by our own knowledge, missing out on valuable insights from those around us, and making unwise health decisions.[6]

The Importance of Health Humility

Health humility is a learning, open-minded mindset that allows us to question and seek out information. We've lost the art of health humility and have become health arrogant. Health arrogance is the inflated sense of knowledge and understanding about your health and what impacts it. We all struggle with health arrogance. I think it's because it's easier to justify what we do (or don't do) after the fact than to do the work before we act. We think we can outsmart our biology without truly

continued

understanding it. So, we choose the easy option or the biology hack. We ignore our symptoms, are easily persuaded to try random approaches, believe lies about our health when we shouldn't, and don't believe truths when we should.

Other cultures revere health as part of their identity, recognizing the possibilities of healing rather than just treating illness. We in the U.S. need to adopt this mindset to stop seeing health as something separate from us and start embracing it as part of who we are. Health is not a destination; it's a way of being Health is not something to manage, like our bills, it's a part of who we are. We must begin to nurture, not treat, our health.

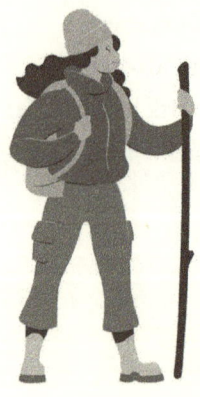

Health humility opens the door to new healing possibilities.

Humility is a superpower—it is a strength, not a weakness. Humility leads us to recognize that we don't have all the answers, and that's okay. Recognizing the importance of humility in our health journey, we embark on a path of exploration and guidance-seeking. We are committed to perpetual learning and ongoing self-education. By staying open to new knowledge and experiences, we ensure that we never hinder our own progress on the road to better health. You, my friend, are already showing that you have health humility by embarking on the Health Hero journey. You are a rare find and I am honored you are here!

The Surreptitious Seven

Here is a recap of the Surreptitious Seven. I suggest you revisit this list whenever considering a major health decision to make sure you're not falling into one of these traps.

- **Reacting to health scares:** waiting until a problem arises instead of preventing it
- **Ignoring body signals:** overlooking early signs until they escalate
- **Emotional decision-making:** letting emotions cloud health choices
- **Becoming overwhelmed by information:** struggling to filter out noise from helpful health advice
- **Overlooking alternatives:** not exploring options beyond the doctor's office
- **Lacking a strategic evaluation:** failing to track progress and adjust efforts
- **Lacking health humility:** believing we know it all, closing ourselves off to new insights

The Curiosity Cure

No matter which or how many of the Surreptitious Seven tendencies you identified with, there's a unifying thread that weaves through the countermeasures, a thread we must acknowledge and rekindle: **our lost curiosity**. Somewhere along the way, in the busyness of life and the noise of the world, we have lost our innate curiosity about ourselves and our health. It's too easy to take a pill when something hurts or ignore a symptom altogether.

In my thirty years of helping clients, I've seen firsthand how curiosity accelerates healing. When my clients explored multiple modalities—whether supplements, nutrition changes, or movement—they found the best interventions for their unique needs.

We need curiosity to drive ourselves to want to learn more: more about why we're overweight, why we feel sluggish, why we can't eat this food or that without getting an upset stomach. We also must question the norms and conventional wisdom surrounding health practices. Why do people these days not cook their dinner? Why is it that fast food tastes so good, yet it makes us feel sluggish after we eat it?

If we want to live longer, better lives, we must become explorers again. We need to take back our curiosity, apply it to our health, and use it as a tool for logic and reason. That's how we break the current paradigm. That's how we survive.

Dive into a world of learning and actively seek fresh perspectives on health management. Find books, videos, articles, and ask healthier people about their perspectives. Engage in thought-provoking discussions and participate in workshops or seminars. Embark on an exhilarating quest for knowledge.

Our health doesn't happen to us—it's something we must discover, question, nurture, and embrace. And it all starts with curiosity. You are now stepping into your role as a Health Hero—ready to navigate the challenges, take charge of your well-being, and inspire those around you. You must change your thinking in order to change your health.

Don't be afraid to step into uncharted territories of managing your health but observe how each new intervention influences your health and well-being. Be curious about you and how your body reacts to things. Decipher your body's language—what is it telling you? I help you translate your body's signals in later chapters. This curiosity-driven approach shifts you from being set in a way that you think is right to one that your body tells you is right. This curiosity-driven transformation shifts you from passive health management to an active, informed journey of exploration, questioning, and experimentation, ultimately leading to a holistic and personalized approach to recovery and health.

Empowering Your Health Hero

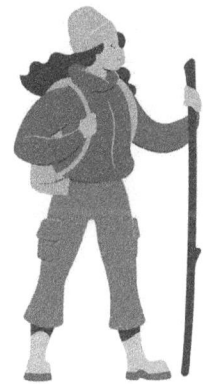

You now know the enemies getting in the way of your health and making good health decisions. You are also now armed with humility and curiosity. This means that you're willing to learn new things and step outside what you've done before to manage your health (but leaning on what you know works to help your health, too). And you're more curious than ever to listen to what your body is saying, question why things are the way they are, why you do what you do, and if what you're hearing in the wild is really true when it comes to managing your health. You'll also become more open to trying new approaches to manage your health—ones you never would have considered before. You're ready. Healing potential waits, so let's find it together.

> Curiosity releases opportunities only if a person lets it.

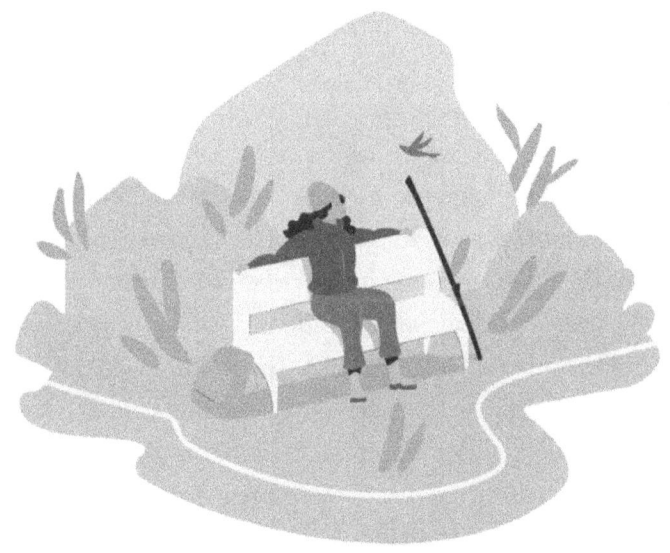

CHAPTER 2

Recognizing Thinking That May Be Holding You Back

I f you're up against a health challenge, grab your curiosity and take a health humility pill because you're going to need to humble yourself and be willing to open your eyes to the thinking traps that might be preventing you from reaching your health and healing potential. This is where Health Heroes transform from stuck to healed.

One of the most memorable scenes from *The Empire Strikes Back* is where Yoda tells Luke Skywalker that he can use the Force to lift his X-wing fighter from the swamp where it is mired. Luke says, "I'll give it a try," and Yoda replies, "Do. Or do not. There is no try." Luke fails the test, and the fighter slides deeper into the muck. Then Yoda raises the fighter. One of the lessons from the scene is that Luke failed because he did not believe he could perform the task. His thinking limited his achievements.

As Luke learned on his path to becoming a Jedi master, often our greatest adversaries hide within us. It's not a supervillain or a sinister force, but subtle biases and mental shortcuts can cloud our judgment, steering us off course when we least expect it. And the scariest part of it all is that we are totally unaware that we're being led astray.

Limiting beliefs go beyond not thinking we are capable of doing something, like what happened to Luke. The fact is, we are all bound to the limits of our thinking: we only know what we know, and until and unless we seek new knowledge, we're limited by our current knowledge. That is why, as I discuss in the previous chapter, curiosity is so important when it comes to managing our health—it allows us to ask questions and opens the door to learning new information.

The catch-22 here is that we all have a hard time recognizing self-limiting beliefs in ourselves because we are limited in our thinking! This is where health humility comes in—you must be willing to recognize, or at least admit, that you have limiting beliefs that are getting in the way of your best health.

Maybe you believe that your genetics have predetermined certain health conditions and there's nothing you can do to change that. Or perhaps a doctor once told you that you would have a health issue for the rest of your life, and now you're convinced you'll never fully be well. These beliefs can feel like hard truths, but they often aren't the whole story. Yes, genetics and chronic conditions play a role, but they don't define your entire health journey. There are countless interventions and proactive choices you can make that can positively impact your health—often in ways you might not expect.

I've seen it time and time again with my clients, whether they were battling skin issues, chronic fatigue, digestive disorders, or hormonal imbalances. The biggest breakthrough wasn't just in finding the right treatment—it was in overcoming their own limited thinking. So don't be surprised if you, too, find yourself grappling with self-imposed barriers as you work to improve your health.

I'll say it again because it's that important: you will, guaranteed, encounter one continual obstacle over and over again when you're working through a health issue—yourself. The more you recognize yourself as the obstacle, the better you'll become at mastering your thinking, and each time you do, you'll expand your healing potential and become more efficient at recovering from health concerns.

This chapter is designed to help you understand the limits of your beliefs that may make it harder to achieve health or fitness goals. Let's experience the profoundly impactful motivations behind what you *don't* know. I've put together some of the most common limiting beliefs that I've seen get in the way of my clients' best health. As you read through this list, ask yourself (and be honest!) if you have found yourself subject to them now or at one time or another. Remember, be kind to yourself—this is an exercise in curiosity, not a finger-pointing session. Health humility opens the door to doing better, and it's the way we become a true Health Hero.

Limited Thinking Leads to Limited Healing

In our journey toward better health, our mindset can either propel us forward or hold us back. Often, limited thinking clouds our decision-making, keeping us stuck in our current health status. Thoughts like "I'm not enthusiastic or excited about being intentional about my health, so it's

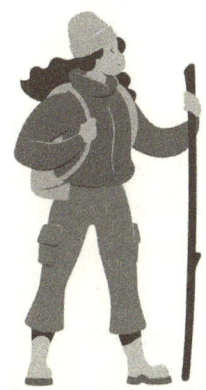

Check yourself before you wreck yourself.

really not that important to me," or "I don't have enough time to focus on my health—I'm too busy," are common barriers we place in our own way. Even the belief that "I'm already doing everything I can to heal or to be healthy" can prevent us from exploring new possibilities for improvement. It's time to address head-on the most common three limiting thoughts and how to overcome them. See if you recognize yourself in any of these thoughts.

Thought 1: I'm not enthusiastic or excited about being intentional about my health, so it's really not that important to me. Is it really that health isn't important to you, or is it that taking care of your health will take too much time or work, or be unrewarding or tedious?

For people with this self-limiting belief, the idea of taking care of their health day in and day out creates an automatic negative response. True, the journey to better health takes time and energy—just as do other aspects of your life, like cleaning your house, doing your laundry, or getting the oil changed in your car. It's hard to face tasks like this with enthusiasm or excitement. I've never heard of someone exclaim their excitement about cleaning the bathroom, for example. In fact, it's perfectly normal to feel some sense of burden that comes with caring for your health. Could this be why you feel aversion to taking care of your health?

Many of my clients feel the same way when we first meet. Later they get into the routine of addressing their health, begin to feel better, and it becomes an essential part of their day. This will happen to you, too, if you remove the belief that taking good care of yourself is always going to feel miserable or be hard. For example, there will always be reasons to not exercise, but building time to exercise will almost always result in feeling better. Give your body a chance to be healthy by taking healing into your own hands and choosing to do what it takes to be healthy.

Thought 2: I don't have enough time to focus on my health—I'm too busy. If this self-limiting belief is resonating with you, I can relate. I'm busy, too. But it's wrong to think that you don't have time to be healthy—we make the time for the things that are most important to us, or that make us feel good. Look at your discretionary time—what is it that you do during that time? The thing you do the most is the thing you prioritize. Is it something that numbs your thinking, like movies or TV, or video games or social media? Whatever it is, what is it about that thing that appeals most to you? The limiting belief here is that time is the enemy, but the truth is that you haven't prioritized health in the top things to spend your time on. Why is that? What is it that is keeping you from spending time on your health? Is it the previous limiting belief that it will be too hard? Or is it that you don't know where to begin? Be curious, ask yourself why, and don't judge. We create the limiting belief, so we can overcome it, too—we just need to be honest and patient with ourselves.

Thought 3: I'm already doing everything I can to heal (an ailment) or to be healthy. Does this limiting belief resonate with you? The truth is that none of us are doing everything possible. That is why I wrote this book. You may be doing your best, but that's different. May I respectfully say that your best can be better? Thinking that doing everything you can is good enough is a self-limiting belief. Our thoughts are limiting, remember? There's always more we can do, always different approaches we can try—and the options are limitless. That doesn't mean you're not doing a good job at managing your health. You may already be a Health Hero. But even the strongest of Health Heroes needs to learn, grow, and try new ways to stay healthy and heal.

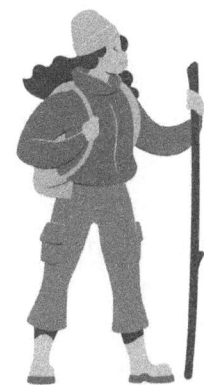

Healing starts with your thinking.

Additionally, what used to work in the past won't always translate to the future, so continuing to do what we've already done will not guarantee improvement or success in the future. Our health and bodies are constantly changing, and, as such, our approach should be changing with it. We aren't doing everything; we're doing something, and we can do more. But some of you might be satisfied with how you feel and how you approach your health. At some point you won't be satisfied, guaranteed, so when that time comes, this book will be waiting. For everyone else, these are exciting times because there are new ways to heal and take care of our health waiting for us, right now.

Did you recognize yourself in any of these self-limiting beliefs? If you do, then challenge yourself to think about where your self-limiting belief comes from and how it's *preventing* you from achieving your best health.

How Biases Blind You from Options

Education, experience, knowledge, upbringing, intelligence—none of these serve as an adequate predictor as to why one person makes one type of health decision while another makes an entirely different decision when they are presented with similar situations and information. What is going on behind the scenes that no one seems to understand?

Part of the answer has to do with how our brains make decisions. The gap that exists between making a good health decision and a not-so-good one is often filled by biases. Biases are a specific form of limited thinking brought about by our brain's attempt to simplify our decisions. This helpful, built-in brain tool saves our brain time and energy. But sometimes the leaps in logic leave us lagging in health.[1]

Biases also allow us to make shortcuts to alleviate overthinking and cognitive distress. For example, humans have an innate inclination toward instant gratification, often referred to as **present bias**. This is why we choose the donut, which offers immediate pleasure, over the salad whose benefits lie in the future. It also makes sense why many of us choose the fix-it-now approach instead of stopping to think about what the best choice *really* is for our long-term health. Present bias threatens our future health.

Add to present bias a sales marketing strategy from a health sales industry trying to persuade you to buy or try their health-reversing amazing product. You're already prone to present bias, so add to that a clever sales pitch and voilà—you have a bad health decision in the making. I'm not saying that these decisions will always be detrimental or will forever impact your health (although they might be), but poor decisions cost us time, money, and effort—they are an inefficiency when it comes to healing.

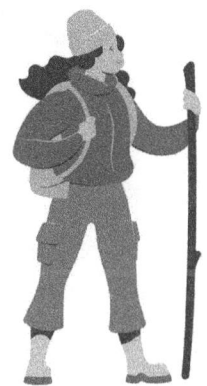

Present bias threatens our **future** health.

Your Health Is for Sale. It's Time to Take It off the Market.

Marketers are very savvy about how to present their messages in ways that connect with us emotionally. Even though we know their intent is to get us to purchase something, their messages can sneak past our defenses. This is especially true if the advertising includes powerful visual images. We humans are, after all, primarily visual creatures (half of our brain's resources are dedicated to seeing and interpreting what we see). Who among us doesn't want to have the same life as the happy, beautiful, skinny people enjoying a fulfilling life that we see in the ads? Businesses make millions of dollars using marketing knowledge, and the beauty and well-being sales industry is in the business of making money, so they are no different. They don't want what's best for your overall health, they want you

continued

> to buy their product. The next time you see a sales pitch for a supplement or health improvement program, put aside your temptation to be persuaded and step into your Health Hero mentality and ask yourself, "Is this really true?" The reality is, what you see portrayed in the marketing messages is seldom what you'll see in results for yourself.

Present bias can also strongly influence our decisions in the doctor's office. When faced with a health decision, we might be inclined to follow our doctor's advice without fully exploring other options simply because it feels easier and more reassuring at the moment. This can squelch our curiosity about what might truly be the best choice for us, leading us to accept the first solution offered rather than considering alternatives that could better align with our needs and preferences.

To address present bias in the moment, it's important to pause and reflect before making a decision. Ask yourself questions like, "Am I choosing this because it feels like the quickest solution?" or "Have I explored all my options?" By taking a step back and allowing yourself time to think critically, you can balance the immediate comfort of following the doctor's advice with the long-term benefits of making a decision that's truly right for you. Additionally, consider seeking a second opinion or doing some research to ensure that the path you're choosing is the best fit for your health goals.

Back to biases: Although our biased, limiting thinking is part of our human nature, we rarely recognize biases in ourselves unless we're looking for them, and yet we are quick to see them in others. This is called the **bias blind spot**. To help us see that we can overcome limited thinking (but never entirely), I've put together a list of eight of the most common biases that I've encountered with my clients. Can you name a time when you have succumbed to any of these naughty biases?

1) Anchoring bias: This bias occurs when we anchor our perspective heavily on some form of initial information. We then place too much value on this initial information, which then influences our future health decisions. This bias was obviously prevalent when the pandemic hit the country. Some people were convinced they should get vaccinated, while others were convinced to do the opposite. When I asked people which information they heard first, in almost every case, the first protocol they heard was the one they chose to follow. Be careful; what you hear first is what you'll gravitate toward choosing later on. Anchoring bias locks us into a set path, rather than tuning us into the facts and reality of the situation. Make sure that what you choose is the *best* choice, regardless of if it was the first choice.

2) Bandwagon effect: The bandwagon effect refers to the tendency we have to adopt certain behaviors, styles, or attitudes simply because everyone else is doing it. In terms of health, I see this play out in many ways. A diet or fitness plan is chosen because everyone else is following it, or we eat the same thing other people eat because it's the thing to do at the time—"When in Paris." Look for times when you're tempted to follow the crowd when it's not healthy. Do what you need to do to maintain your best health, regardless of if you're going along with the crowd or not. This takes some practice because social pressure is incredibly powerful.

3) Bounded rationality: Bounded rationality refers to the idea that in decision-making, we are limited by the information we have, the ways in which our brain processes information, and the finite amount of time we have to make decisions. In the context of health, this means that we might not make the optimal health choices, because we are working with limited knowledge, resources, or understanding.

For example, a person who chooses a particular health intervention based on the limited information available to them, rather than the most effective or comprehensive option, is experiencing bounded rationality. They might decide to take a popular over-the-counter medication for their symptoms without fully understanding its side effects or without exploring more effective treatments due to time constraints or limited access to better information.

If you're reading this, you are already overcoming the limits of your bounded rationality by expanding your perspective.

I run across bounded rationality in people who are practicing extreme health management practices (like intense exercise programs or extreme diets) and have rigid rules they follow around their health. They believe the limits of their practices are all they need to follow to be healthy. I also see this play out when people are overconfident about how they're managing their health, and there are apparent outward signs that they are not making as many good choices as they think they are. In other words, sometimes we think we're doing a great job managing an aspect of our health, but it's obvious we're not. We are and forever will be bound by our rationality because we'll never know everything there is to know. But the more we learn, the more we will begin to recognize there is always more to learn about our health and how to manage it. We should never stop learning and breaking through bounded rationality!

4) Decision fatigue: If you've ever had to make a decision after making multiple prior decisions, you likely experienced this bias. Or if you have too many options, like when staring down an aisle with dozens of options of supplements, decision fatigue sets in and you pick one based on a single criterion (studies show that it's strongly associated with the visual element on the package—surprise!).[2] We then further justify the decision by saying it was cheaper, looked like it was trustworthy, sounded appealing, was "good enough," etc. Some people experience decision fatigue and simply don't make a decision, because it's too mentally exhausting. When this happens, take a break and later focus on the most important elements of the product you need. Do some research, which I show you how to do in later chapters, so you can be assured you're making a good decision instead of a haphazard one.

5) Dunning–Kruger effect: Put most simply, this bias describes our ability to overestimate our knowledge and competence in areas we haven't studied or been trained in. It is named after two researchers, Justin Kruger and David Dunning. It's easy to let this bias creep in and show itself when we get puffed up in thinking we know more than we do or when we downplay what we really know and don't think we know as much as we do. It's a fine line between being in tune with what we know and what we don't know. We must be honest with ourselves when facing our health knowledge. From there, we can seek more knowledge to fill in the gaps.

A good example of the Dunning–Kruger effect in the context of managing health is when an individual with minimal knowledge or experience in nutrition believes they are an expert. For instance, someone might read a few articles or watch a couple of videos about diet and nutrition and then confidently start advising others on what they should eat or what supplements they should take. Despite their lack of in-depth understanding, they may dismiss advice from actual health professionals, thinking they know better. This overconfidence in their limited knowledge can lead to poor health decisions, such as adopting fad diets or taking unnecessary supplements, which might not only be ineffective but potentially harmful.

6) Status quo bias: Status quo bias is the tendency to prefer things to stay the same rather than change. In the context of health, this can manifest as a reluctance to adopt new health practices or treatments, even if they might be beneficial. People with status quo bias might stick to their existing routines and habits simply because they are familiar and comfortable, rather than because they are the best choices for their health.

Keeping our health situation the same, despite evidence that the opposite is needed, is how we can spot this bias. When I worked in the field of cardiac rehabilitation, I had patients who were content with their health until the big heart attack event. Many of them knew that they were at a high risk for a cardiac event, but they were content doing what they always did despite that knowledge. On one hand, this approach could be viewed as contentment. "I'm fine this way." But for the Health Hero who is looking to overcome ailments, there is no room for status quo bias because we are always continuing to learn and expand our knowledge and try new approaches to manage our health.

I've also had clients think that doing what they've always done will automatically get them new results. It took me a while to recognize this as status quo bias. They were settled in their behavior and really weren't ready to change. As the saying goes, "If you do what you've always done, you'll get what you always have gotten." The difference is that Health Heroes are ready to change and be proactive when it comes to their health. They're not passive, they're active. They're continually tweaking and modifying their health approach because they recognize that their bodies are always shifting and dynamic. I talk more about this in later chapters.

7) Sunk cost fallacy: It's hard to give up something we've put so much effort into, even if it's apparent that what we're doing isn't working. When it comes to our health, this bias shows up when we spend lots of time or money on an attempt to get healthier. We're tenacious but not rational when we decide that we're not going to give up trying this effort, because of the cost we've already sunk into it.

I have fallen prey to this fallacy many times. I sunk hundreds of dollars into essential oils and supplements, thinking that they were doing something for me, when in reality I didn't see any measurable impact. I refused to stop because I had invested so much in it. Finally, after learning more about biases, I realized it was time to stop the madness. It was like fishing when there were no fish to be had. I cut the bait and let it go. I had fished enough for evidence and there wasn't any. I now track my interventions to verify measurable impact and so I give it enough time to be certain it's worthwhile. I teach you to do this, too, later in the book.

8) No-fail assumption: I collect self-help books that I constantly reference. It's also kind of a hobby of mine. Many of my books offer a method, a strategy, an approach that is insightful and likely helpful when applied. But others are hilarious and offer up the most nonsensical approaches to being young, getting a booty like twenty-year-old model, or improving your brain to become an Einstein. Based on the collective wisdom from the books I have on my shelf, I theoretically could live to 300 thanks to the promise of reversing the aging process.

How in the world do we ever fall prey to thinking we can reverse aging? Biases and limited thinking are to blame! It may be ludicrous, but we really do think we can reverse aging by reading a book and following their advice!

I actually love these books because they remind me of the empty promises that we are prone to buy into. They are the examples of how biases can potentially get us to do the craziest of health endeavors. I'd give you an example, but you would be tempted to try it because that's how powerful the messaging in these books can be.

The reality is that there is always another side to the promise these books and health programs try to sell us. And there's always another side to our perception of the problem. Nothing can be promised because everything is a process. We oversee how much we want to try to improve—that is what we can control. I call this psychological control—we have a lot of power in controlling how we think. There are also physical aspects that we must consider as well—physical control—which I cover later.

But I want you to remember this: **you will never find one approach to your health that is free from errors or that guarantees that you won't ever get sick or age.** And we will always be subject to misjudgment. It's part of being human. And not all mistakes are bad—mistakes teach us. And there is no fail-safe way to approach your health but this one—do your best. That is exactly what you are doing now by reading this book. Your best just got better by understanding how flawed thinking can give you a false perception of being right.

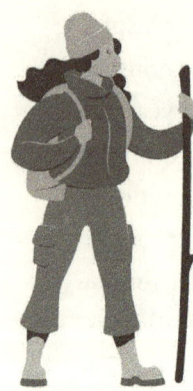

Untether Your Thinking

> Our thinking is the ceiling to our healing.

There is a universal truth that we can't fix a problem until we recognize it. That's why, as I said before, awareness is the best and perhaps only antidote for biases. We don't have to fight the battle against self-limiting beliefs or biases—we just need to recognize when biases might be getting in the way of progress and healing. If you see yourself in any of the descriptions I provide in this chapter, challenge yourself to consider options or information beyond the borders you've erected around your thinking.

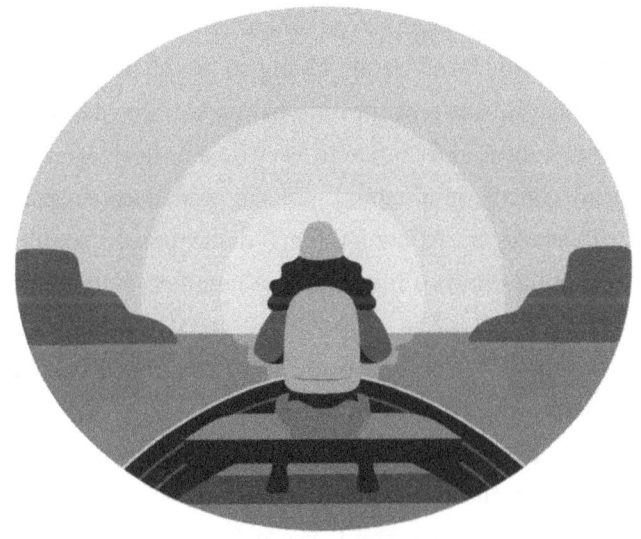

CHAPTER 3

Swimming Upstream in the Culture Current

Every single human on this planet lives within a culture, the collective beliefs and habits of the people that surround them. Yet in the hustle and bustle of our daily lives, it's rare that we pause to contemplate how out culture affects our health decisions, for better or worse. Instead, we go about our routines, often oblivious to the subtle ways in which our surroundings, our communities, and our upbringing have shaped our perspectives on well-being and our day-to-day health decisions.

It's as if we're carried along by an invisible current, following the norms and practices established by our cultural milieu and the people who inhabit it. Rarely do we question these influences, let alone challenge them. Yet, our health is intricately entwined with the culture that surrounds us. It's time to practice the skill of awareness of how connected your culture is to your well-being. Doing so gives you the keys to navigate diverse health intervention options, make informed choices that align with your values, and craft your very own health narrative.

During my time in graduate school, my ambitions took a sporting turn. As I observed my fellow students' dedication to training, I was inspired to adopt a rigorous lifestyle, involving heavy weightlifting and regular running and cycling. I keenly observed my body transform, watching my muscles grow, and soon, I too felt myself becoming lean and mean, thanks to their ultra-fit influence.

However, a sense of unease began to creep in. Despite my newfound agility and lean physique, I noticed something was amiss. Lifting my arms for longer than a few seconds was exhausting, and easy hikes left me surprisingly drained. I also became less flexible. In response, I worked out harder and more often.

Over a span of two years, I began to gradually recognize a significant shift in my perspective. Despite being immersed in a community of athletes and feeling the pressure to keep up, I came to the realization that my desire wasn't merely about winning races or competitions. What truly mattered to me was placing a higher emphasis on my physical well-being with a compassionate and sustainable approach. Looking back, I wish I had been more attuned to the cultural forces influencing my health decisions. If I had understood that the lifestyle I had embraced didn't align with my overall well-being and personality, I could have charted my unique path to a healthier life much earlier.

Nevertheless, I wouldn't alter a single aspect of that journey, because it proved to be a priceless learning experience. It provided me with invaluable insights into tailoring physical activity to suit both my personal preferences and my body's unique needs. No matter where you've been on your health journey, your experiences are equally invaluable.

They serve as a guide, helping you to identify the approaches that benefit you and those that don't. In this chapter, I talk about how you evaluate the positive and negative impacts that culture may be having on your health decisions.

Cultivating Health Perspectives: Unraveling the Concept of Culture

Taking one step back, let's define culture. What is culture, anyway? I'm reminded of my time in the microbiology lab, where I nurtured minuscule bacterial organisms in petri dishes, creating the perfectly warm, dark, and humid conditions for their growth. It was fascinating to observe how these bacteria multiplied and thrived in their designated environment, or didn't, depending on the environmental conditions.

In many ways, our social culture mirrors this microbial growth. The environment in which we are raised and surrounded by offers us valuable social nutrients. However, it's crucial to recognize that not all cultures are beneficial for our well-being. Just as placing bacteria in an unsuitable environment can hinder their growth and vitality, being immersed in a negative cultural context can have a measurable impact on our physical and psychological health, causing distress rather than flourishing.

Yet, the converse is also true—we can not only survive but thrive, even growing stronger amid adverse environments, much like a super bacterium. We can develop resilience and strength when faced with challenging environments, just like super bacteria evolve to overcome antibiotics. Our personal growth and adaptation in the face of adversity is like the way these bacteria build resistance, making us more resilient and capable. To do this, we must first be aware of the impact of negative culture on our health behavior and decisions.

The degree to which we hold our cultural beliefs in high regard plays a pivotal role in determining the extent of influence our culture exerts on us and our health. It's a natural tendency for us to adapt our behavior in alignment with the cultural norms and values we prioritize. Additionally, we constantly engage in comparisons with individuals both within and outside our primary cultural sphere, evaluating our position in this broader context. This ongoing process shapes our perspective on what we perceive as "right" or "best," drawing from the cues and standards set by those around us.

We navigate a multitude of social groups, spanning from vast entities like the nation we reside in down to the intimate circle of friends and family. Each of these cultural spheres exerts its unique influence on us, encompassing both positive and negative aspects that shape our approach to health decision-making.

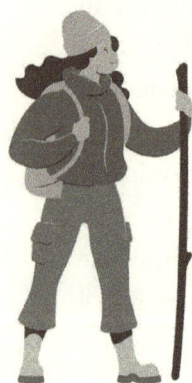

The tribe's pull may be strong, but awareness will help prevent you from just riding along.

Some cultures we inherit have a profound and enduring impact, while others may only leave a fleeting impression, affecting us for mere moments or hours. By sniffing out clues that indicate cultural and social influences, we gain the necessary perspective to ensure our health choices align with our genuine desires and requirements for optimal well-being. Remember, you are the hound, eagerly wagging your tail at the delightful positive influences while letting out a low growl at the cunning negative ones.

Unmasking the U.S. Health Culture

In America, many people treat symptoms without identifying the underlying cause. Although insurance covers more preventive services than it did even ten years ago, it still rarely covers complementary approaches to health management, such as massages and acupuncture.

But health insurance, as it was originally created, was designed to financially cover people in case of illness, not to keep illness from occurring. Although many people are troubled by their health insurance company's lack of coverage when it comes to services such as complementary interventions, I take the stance that we are expecting round pegs to fit square holes when we think of preventive service coverage and insurance. Within other realms of insurance, we don't expect coverage for similar things. For example, our homeowner's coverage doesn't pay for additions to our house to make it sturdier, like storm shutters. Some insurance companies may offer premium discounts to homeowners who have them, but they don't pay for them. Why then would we expect the healthcare system to cover all of the preventive services that can keep us healthy? Perhaps we long for a world where everyone is generous and not out to make a profit, but that just isn't the case, especially when it comes to insurance in general. However, I have hope that someday they will consider covering more services that prevent conditions.

Instead, I recommend that we should be ready to spend some time, energy, and yes, money, to keep ourselves healthy because it should be a priority in our lives. Where we spend our money indicates what we value most and what our priorities are. For example, someone who values socializing and eating out will spend more on dining and entertainment, while someone who values health will happily spend on a gym membership, personal training, and massages. We put our money where our priorities are.

Again, we are not a society that embraces staying well. We are a society that focuses on what to do when we are sick. Doctors are also not well situated to discuss how to prevent an illness; they aren't extensively trained to do so, nor do they have the time (with a few exceptions, like functional medicine providers). Also, one appointment is hardly

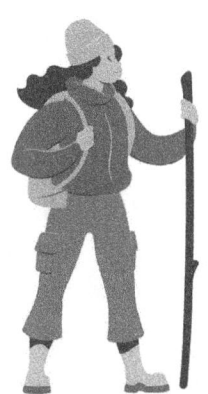

Doctors don't have to treat what we prevent.

enough to work through the best approach to health prevention for each of their patients.

Imagine if you made a doctor's appointment for a preventive visit, and when you got there you said, "Hi Doctor, can I pick your brain on a few alternative options on how to prevent dementia (or whatever you choose) and what to do to keep it away going forward?" (I've not heard of any visits like this, but if you had one, please share how effective it was, and how costly.) We mainly search the internet for such information. Doctors are not bad for not helping us with prevention—they're just focused on their job to treat illness, not prevent it. Regardless, no matter how we approach prevention or treatment, the truth is, we'll pay now on things that keep us healthy or pay later into the healthcare system.

Are Medical Disclaimers Robbing Us of Our Power?

There's one more pervasive aspect of medical care in the U.S. that influences many of our decisions: medical disclaimers. We see these warnings everywhere, urging us to seek the advice of a physician or other qualified healthcare provider before starting an exercise program, trying a new diet, or addressing any health concern on our own. As a result, we've become conditioned to believe we need medical advice for everything, turning us into overly cautious scaredy-cats when it comes to our health.

Don't get me wrong—it's entirely reasonable to consult a doctor when you're facing a significant health issue or need guidance on the safety of medications. But for healthy adults, do we really need to check with a doctor before every decision, like starting an exercise program? Of course not. We are capable adults who can make informed decisions about our health without feeling the need to seek approval for every step we take. Constantly checking in with our doctor takes away our power to manage our health. We've built a doctor-dependent health culture in the U.S., but what we truly need is a self-reliant health culture, where doctors serve as valuable support rather than the driving force behind every decision.

Your Upbringing Matters

Understanding the broader U.S. health culture provides valuable insight into the collective attitudes and behaviors that shape how we manage our health. However, our health decisions are also profoundly influenced by more personal factors—specifically, our upbringing. The values, habits, and beliefs instilled in us from a young age play a crucial role in shaping our approach to health and wellness. This matters because these early influences impact our health decisions and behaviors today—no matter how old you are.

What did you eat growing up? Did your parents cook dinner, did they avoid cooking, or were they somewhere in between? What did their actions tell you about how they valued food? Did they embrace healthy foods, or did they avoid them, or a little of both? From the time that we were very young, we had little control over what we ate. We were at the mercy of our caregivers, and in those formative years we began to get set in our approach to not just food, but in how we were going to see and manage our health.

Then, as we grew older, we began to have some choices about what we wanted to eat. What did you eat when you were growing up and then throughout high school? What did your friends eat? Each social interaction imparted an imprint into how we manage our health today. Maybe we overcame some of the negative tendencies left from our youth, maybe not. Can you identify where you adopted health behaviors when you were younger that you still practice today?

One prime example is eating around the table. When I was growing up, my family traditionally ate dinner every night around a table, and my spouse experienced the same. We passed this behavior to our kids. As they married and had their own families, their spouses brought in their own expectations about eating dinner, and so some traditions were passed, and others were dropped.

Most of the time this occurs without formality—it just happens. Knowing that it happens at all, passing what we learned to our kids, can help you decide if it might be time to change a behavior that has been unhealthy. You can improve your health, and your family's, one positive change at a time.

Who We Hang Around Matters

Our upbringing undeniably shapes our foundational health beliefs and behaviors.[1] Yet, as we move through different stages of life, the influence of our immediate social circles—such as our workplace, friends, and acquaintances—becomes increasingly significant. These small groups of culture create environments that can either support or hinder our health goals. In the following section, we examine how these social networks impact our health decisions and behaviors, illustrating the powerful role of our daily interactions and relationships in our overall well-being.

We encounter small groups of cultures in our neighborhoods, workplaces, places of worship, recreational clubs, sport teams, friends, and even on social media. Each of these distinct groups carries its own set of norms and expectations regarding lifestyle choices, from the food they eat, physical activity they do, and other health-impacting behaviors like drinking, smoking, or vaping.

Each set of social groups has the potential to lead us to a type of bias called **groupthink** that isn't discussed in earlier chapters because I want to bring it up now. Groupthink is a shared sense of reality. Hang around smokers and you'll begin to resonate with their smoking, and you may even start to relate to the smoking logic. The same is true for people who are healthy—they have their own language and approach that is contagious, and eventually you may even start to adopt those behaviors. People are wired for imitation and bond when they're sharing experiences. Who we hang around with and what we're doing when we hang around them matters more than we realize.

We pick up on the behaviors of those around us through our eyes—not necessarily through words. MRI research shows that our brain neurons fire in the very same regions of the brain as those who are actually performing the action—all we need to do is watch. Neurons firing in response to someone else's actions are called mirror neurons, and these visual connections to our brain can help us perform better at sports or arts simply by watching others succeed. Social media is another example—watch a video of someone combing their hair repeatedly and you, too, will start to comb your hair in the same way.

How can we use this information to improve our health decisions? If we want to be healthier, we should hang around healthier people. If we want our kids to be healthier, we need to show them how to be healthier and keep them exposed to other groups where health is valued. It's easier to be healthier together.

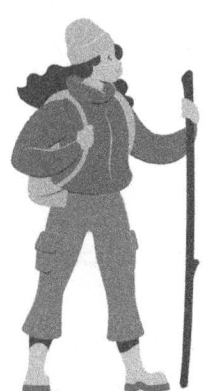

What we see reflects how we think.

What Are Your Cultural Influences?

Understanding the profound impact of social ties and culture on our health behaviors is crucial for making positive adjustments in our lives.[2] To shed light on the ways our family heritage and contemporary tribes shape our health decisions, both positively and negatively, consider these thought-provoking questions:

- What does my heritage say about my identity and values, and how does it affect my approach to health management?
- What healthcare philosophies align with my cultural beliefs?
- What does my culture believe about healing?
- How do stories, art, or traditions influence my health perspectives and practices?
- To what extent do my core beliefs drive my health management choices?
- Who are the key influencers shaping my deeper beliefs, whether they be family, friends, experts, etc.? How much sway do they hold over my behaviors?
- In what ways does the healthcare system contrast with my cultural beliefs, and how does this discrepancy affect me?
- What steps can I take to minimize the negative impact of external influences on my health decisions?

By contemplating these questions, we can gain valuable insights into our cultural and social influences, enabling us to make more informed and health-conscious choices. Once more, keep in mind that your goal is to be like an eager hound, joyfully wagging your tail in response to delightful positive influences and emitting a low growl at the sly negative ones. It's time to call out the negative influences and defend ourselves from their impact.

Navigating the delicate balance between our individual values and the prevailing cultural influences is undoubtedly a challenge. To successfully tread this path, we must sharpen our self-awareness, particularly when it comes to our natural inclination to align with the behaviors of those in our social circles. It's essential to maintain clarity and stay focused on our health objectives, making decisions that align with these intentions, rather than simply conforming to the expectations of others, especially if those expectations don't align with healthy choices.

However, it's equally vital to remain open-minded when those around us genuinely have our best interests at heart and offer different perspectives on health. While their input can be valuable, it's essential to evaluate it in the context of our own knowledge and understanding, appreciating the information without feeling compelled to adopt it if it doesn't align with our health goals. This nuanced approach allows us to strike a balance between our individual values and the influence of our social and cultural surroundings.

Never underestimate your capacity to be a force for positive change in the lives of those around you, particularly if you are a woman, as women often serve as the primary health coordinators for their families. Women possess a unique ability to influence the well-being of those close to them and are more likely to engage in consultations within their inner circles. This places women in a remarkable position; they bear significant caregiver responsibilities while being profoundly influenced by their social surroundings.

Health Heroes in the Home

Women often play a central role in influencing the health culture of the home.[3] They are frequently the primary caregivers, responsible for making healthcare decisions for children, spouses, and sometimes elderly parents, which gives them significant influence over the health practices and habits within the household. Studies have shown that women are more likely to schedule doctor's appointments, manage medications, and ensure family members receive preventive care. According to the National Partnership for Women & Families, women make approximately 80 percent of healthcare decisions for their families.[4]

Additionally, women often take on the role of planning and preparing meals, directly impacting the nutritional health of household members. Research indicates that women's choices in food shopping and meal preparation significantly influence their families' dietary habits.[5] Women are also more likely to seek out health information and share it with their family members, acting as health educators within their households.[6]

Women's health behaviors, such as exercise routines, dietary habits, and preventive care practices, serve as models for other family members, with children in particular likely to adopt the health behaviors demonstrated by their mothers. Additionally, women frequently provide emotional and psychological support to their family members, crucial for mental health and well-being, which can encourage healthier lifestyles and better adherence to medical advice.

Even though women are a key health influencer in the home, they're also under constant pressure to maintain the culture's unrealistic standards when it comes to weight. In my experience, even women who aren't overweight are often battling body image issues and unhealthy relationships with food and fitness.

That is why it is so important to promote a healthy perspective on health in general for women. Doing so will shape the health culture of their homes, influencing both immediate and long-term health outcomes for their families. Women have an even greater opportunity to cultivate a culture of health beyond their homes, within tribes and the broader U.S. community. However, the power to create an environment where others can thrive is not exclusive to women; it is a potential that all of us hold.

Q&A WITH ALICE: DECISIONS FOR LOVED ONES

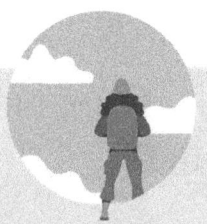

Women carry much of the responsibility for making health decisions for their families or the people they are taking care of. I hear the following question often: "I want to make the best decisions for my family members. How do I know I'm doing that?"

When I was caregiving for family members who were struggling with a health issue, I was given the responsibility of making tough health decisions, and with that came having difficult conversations. It was hard. It would have saved me so much time and angst if I could have had a book to follow so I could check myself and make sure I was looking at all of the angles. What I needed was this book! I needed a process to follow, a way to check if my decisions were on target—a guide to navigating the complex emotions and endless options that come with caregiving. That's exactly what I hope this book becomes for you—a trusted companion on your caregiving journey. In fact, apply all the ideas in this book to your decisions about your loved ones, just as you would do for yourself, and you will know that you've done your best.

Keep on Swimming!

A last bit of advice for all Health Heroes: Because you are choosing a health-conscious lifestyle, those who take a proactive approach to their health might sometimes feel like outsiders within the U.S. culture due to

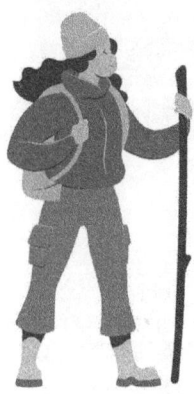

We have power to bring out the best health in those around us.

the prevailing treatment-centered rather than health-forward mindset.

Recognize that embracing a health-oriented lifestyle may feel like swimming upstream and counter to our culture. But be strong, Health Hero, in your identity. Although frustrating, let it fuel your determination to drive positive change within your prevailing culture. In the end, your pursuit of a health-oriented lifestyle will set you apart as a pioneer, paving the way for a healthier future generation.

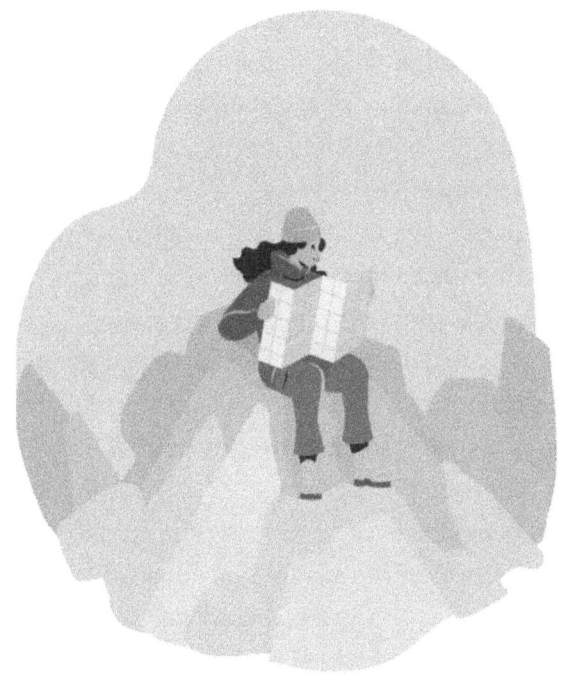

CHAPTER 4

Navigating a Complex Information Landscape

J en was frustrated by her unexplained weight gain over the last four months. She was eating, walking, and exercising the same way as always, yet the scale kept climbing. Jen was on a thyroid replacement medication since she had her thyroid removed a few years ago and suspected it might not be well regulated. But when she had it tested, her thyroid blood levels were normal.

Seeking answers, Jen resolutely sat down to search the internet for why women gain weight in their fifties. She clicked on countless links to various methods for weight loss, from lifestyle changes and cortisol-controlling diets to smoothies and supplements. She found herself going down one rabbit hole after another, seeking out possible reasons why she was gaining weight. She quickly found herself overwhelmed by the sheer volume of conflicting advice.

Finally, Jen landed on a web page that tempted her with the promise of weight loss. All she had to do was pay $200 up front, then $40 a month throughout the three-month program. The program included protein shake powder, a restricted diet protocol, a coach and support group, and online reference resources, like videos. Confident she chose the right option, she purchased the program, awaited her package of protein shake powder, and eagerly set up her account.

The protein powder arrived, and she began consuming it daily, along with following the recommended diet. She connected with her coach and a cohort group and initially began to lose weight. However, around week three, she noticed her energy levels dropping and that she was gaining weight again. Despite sticking to the protocol, her fatigue and weight gain persisted.

Frustrated, she visited her doctor. After new blood work, it was discovered that her thyroid levels had drastically declined. When she explained her weight loss program to her doctor, her doctor quickly identified the issue—the protein shake was interfering with her thyroid medication, causing her thyroid levels to drop, leading to weight gain.

What if Jen had done a quick search to see if the protein shakes would impact her thyroid

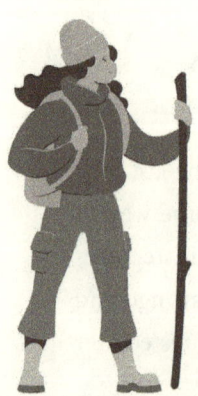

Time spent researching reliable health information BEFORE you choose a path can save you from costly mistakes later.

medication and consulted her doctor before starting the weight loss program? Unfortunately, Jen's venture into the weight loss program cost her time and money. It all could have been avoided with strategic investigation.

Like many of us, Jen ventured unprepared into the vast, often misleading world of the internet. The landscape of online information is like the Wild West—unpredictable, full of twists and turns, and populated with both trustworthy and dubious guides. Who thinks about how their searches today result in personally curated results based on what they've searched for in the past? Knowing that our searches yield more of what the search engines think we want to see risks omitting what else we should know and other options out there.[1] It's easy to see how the internet, with its convenient information at our fingertips, is both an asset and an obstacle.

The truth is, we are all easily persuaded, misinformed, biased, and emotionally charged humans who jump on the internet looking for solutions to our health woes. We need a filter that allows us to search and find what we need without being misled. We also need to know how long to search so that decision fatigue doesn't cloud our judgment. It's past time that we have a game plan to follow as we use the internet for health searches so we can be vigilant and still find the answers we need, and that plan is in the next section.

Where to Begin Your Search on the Internet

I can't tell you how many times I've sat down in front of the computer screen and opened up my search engine and experienced the emotion of hope. Oh, the promise of a fresh online search that will deliver the information I need—it's so close, yet so far. But what happens next is anything but straightforward.

When I'm tired, I notice that my searches are simple descriptions of a symptom: "joints hurt." It's like a primitive cry for someone to just read my mind and figure it out for me. Sometimes I get inspired and detail out a more elaborate search: "knee and ankle stiffness that decreases after several minutes of gentle movement." Which search will give me the best answer? You probably think it's the second one, but the answer is, it depends. The search itself will likely give you a great response somewhere within the literally millions of results, but it's a matter of whether you can find it.

I wish I could give you a step-by-step approach to finding the exact internet information you need to help you solve your health issue. The fact is, I can't, because it's impossible. The best that can be done when searching on the internet is to help you to not be tricked into believing bad information or neglecting to search the other side of the story. You also must consider your uniqueness and unique set of circumstances. But that being the case, I want to provide you with some tips to help you filter good information from the bad so you can get the most of your internet research. Keep these tips by your side as you search for internet health information and check yourself to make sure you've done your best.

Tip #1: Use specific search terms. Use the most precise search terms you can think of. You can even try to put quotes around the term so that results are only what you type—no word within the quotes will be omitted in the search. Change the word order if you don't get the desired results. If you can't define what it is you're searching for, start with broad terms and find other terms to use and start to narrow your search from broad to specific. Remember, someone out there has put specific information on the internet about your very health issue, even perhaps addressing your unique circumstance. The more detailed you get, the more likely you are to find it.

Tip #2: Spend the most time looking at information on quality websites. Find websites that contain information from unbiased resources, such as nonprofit organizations that advocate around health concerns (like the American Heart Association or American Cancer Society), university or government websites, or medical organizations (such as Cleveland Clinic or Mayo Clinic). No matter where you end up,

I've created some criteria to help you identify a high-quality website and high-quality information to make sure it's worth your while (see figure 4.1). For example, pay attention to details like the date of the information to make sure it's still relevant to the times.

Health Information Quality Checklists
Websites

- The information provider, sponsor, and author are clearly identified.
- Disclaimers, conflicts of interest, and limitations are mentioned.
- If commercial interests are present, they are conspicuously declared.
- Links work and are current.
- No unrelated ads are present on the web page.
- Website content has little to no spelling, grammatical, or typographical errors.
- Website administrator or article author contact information is clearly provided.
- Organization or individual mission is available.
- Confidentiality and security are mentioned when giving personal information, including purchase information.
- The information relates directly to the search topic.
- The primary purpose of the website is to provide information, not sell a product or service.
- The website has a current copyright date on the bottom of the web page.
- The website is easy to read, navigate, and easy to use.
- The website is regularly updated, stable, and always accessible.
- The website's purpose is clear (educate, persuade, sell, or entertain).

Information

- Articles and information identify the publish date or dates of posting and the latest updates.
- Content is authoritative and not merely opinionated.
- Content is not intended to promote a product or service.
- Information includes alternative approaches and viewpoints neutrally and with reference justification.
- The purpose of the article is clear.
- Research references are listed.
- Language is clearly written and understandable.
- The audience is clearly identified.
- The author of the information has definitive and easily verifiable qualifications in the subject matter.
- The tone is professional and neutral and not intended to evoke exaggerated emotions.
- Information has been reviewed for accuracy or validated by an expert with extensive knowledge and experience in the trade or profession.

Figure 4.1: Health Information Quality Checklists

Tip #3: Search for academic research papers. Find topics like comparisons of different treatments, information about medication side effects, or how to treat certain health conditions. Reading research papers is a health information secret weapon because research papers break down the issue very concisely in the introduction and tell you what they find in the conclusion. That's right, you don't have to read the whole paper (unless you want to)! Many times, unbiased, trusted websites cite these resources within their article, so they save you the trouble of having to hunt down research papers—just keep an eye out for the references within the website (usually cited in the text and referenced at the bottom of the web page or article).

Use the language you find on the internet or in the research papers to refine your search and start to add in words that address your unique circumstance or needs. One you find the suite of words that suits your situation and is pulling up what you wanted in general, you can begin to add on nuances at the end to refine your search, such as "complementary therapies to help," or "nutrition recommendations," or "things I should consider."

When diving into research, it's crucial to keep an eye out for conflicts of interest—where the researcher may be biased because of what institution they work for or where they get their funding. That information is typically found at the end of research papers. These can reveal whether the study was funded by a pharmaceutical company or other entities that might have a vested interest in the outcome. For instance, reading about a "fabulous" new drug that was researched by the same company selling it should raise a red flag. Instead, look for studies that have undergone solid, unbiased research, ideally conducted across multiple countries. While cultures may differ, humans respond to treatments in similar ways, and international studies help ensure that the findings are more reliable and less influenced by local biases or interests. Always seek out the most objective and comprehensive research to help inform you of your options.

Tip #4: Ask yourself, "What's missing?" Ask yourself some of these questions as you're searching and finding relevant information: What are the essentials I need to know first? What am I missing? What is the negative side of this promise, treatment, or process? What peculiarities exist that make me atypical and that I should consider? Narrow down your searches based on the answers to these questions.

Tip #5: Look at multiple perspectives. Cross-check facts from different reputable sources to ensure you're getting a well-rounded view. Compare what you find with at least two more sources to validate your findings. The weightier the decision, the more sources should be used for validation. Sources besides the internet, such as books, articles, expert opinions, educational videos, or other quality sources can also be used to reinforce your findings.

Consideration of Alternative Sites

I'm going to say something that may surprise you but go ahead and look at information that isn't as reputable *after* you have researched facts. What do sites that are considered "on the fringes" or even "out in left field" by the medical establishment say about the issues you're investigating? Do they promise something that the other websites couldn't? Are they trying to meet a gap that traditional approaches don't have, or are they just trying to capitalize on your condition? What are some comments and feedback people are giving regarding the topic? Are you sensing some reoccurring themes from different sources?

Stand strong and don't buy into empty promises—this is your chance to make sure you're getting your questions answered that traditional resources didn't provide. Take this information into account but be careful to not give it too much weight—just

continued

> include it in the mix of information you want to consider. If you take a lot of time checking out the other side of the story, be sure to make sure you don't get lost in hype. Stay objective, learn, but don't react.

Keeps these tips by your computer as you search the internet for health information so you can keep yourself accountable. Once you use them a few times, you'll be able to search like a Health Hero without them because you'll have the objectivity needed to find what you need, faster.

Using AI to Make Smarter Health Decisions

AI, such as ChatGPT or Claude, or even AI assistants found on your browser, offers a convenient and powerful tool for making more informed, personalized health decisions. It can act like a knowledgeable research assistant, sifting through vast amounts of information to help you explore options, identify possible treatments, or even weigh the pros and cons of different approaches. Think of AI as a starting point to help you gather insights faster and pinpoint strategies that could work for you. But remember, it's a tool to assist in your journey, not to be the "be-all and end-all" voice of health reasoning.

When using AI to explore health options, ask general questions about a condition or treatment you're considering. For instance, if you're curious about alternative therapies for joint pain, AI can summarize research, highlight common approaches, and compare them. The key is to be specific enough to get useful answers while searching creatively by phrasing queries to cover different perspectives. You can then bring this information to your doctor to discuss what fits your unique health situation best.

Use AI with Caution and Curiosity

While AI can guide you toward helpful information, it doesn't know the specifics of your health history or what may be contraindicated for your condition. Use it as a "health navigator" to gather possibilities, but always verify the insights with additional sources, such as your healthcare professional. Keep in mind that privacy matters, too—use caution and don't share personal, sensitive information when using AI, or when using regular search engines like Google. Frame your queries generally or hypothetically to protect your personal health details. AI should spark curiosity, helping you discover what's out there while encouraging a cautious and thoughtful approach.

For a deeper dive into using AI for personal health decisions, including privacy considerations, check out my newsletter article, "AI-Driven Personal Health Decisions." It guides you step-by-step in making an informed, well-considered choice using AI. Use AI as one of many tools in your health tool kit, letting it inspire new possibilities without letting go of your own intuition and professional advice.

What to Do with Health Information from Physicians and Other Healthcare Professionals

As we look to doctors and other healthcare professionals for help and guidance, most would agree that doctors have our best interest in mind. But sometimes, we don't trust our doctor or healthcare provider or their information for one reason or another. This can create a stumbling block to making a good health decision because we omit a source of information to consider. When this happens, remember the following three points, and reconsider considering their information.

1. **Recognize that doctors are human.** Each doctor brings a distinctive package of knowledge, competence, and experience. Each has a unique personality, level of professionalism, credibility, and availability, and no doctor is perfect. When a doctor makes us uncomfortable,

either the way they interact or the information they provide, take that into consideration with the information, and don't necessarily throw the baby out with the bathwater. You can also try voicing concerns and seeing if the patient-doctor relationship can be regained to the point you would consider their information worthwhile. In other words, give them a chance. Who knows if perhaps your physician or healthcare provider was simply having a bad day. If you feel like there's little chance of you feeling comfortable with your doctor or their information, consider getting a second opinion.

2. Evaluate confidence and trust in the doctor. Trust in our doctor matters; the more we trust our doctor, the more likely we will be honest and open with them, and the more likely we will believe the information they provide. And the more we respect our doctor, the more likely we will adhere to their treatment plan. Patient-physician trust is shaped by many factors, such as how both patient and doctor communicate, history with the doctor, and so much more. Do you want to waste any more time with a doctor once that trust is broken? It might be time to find another physician when you don't feel comfortable with the one you have. Don't be afraid to try a remote virtual physician if none are located nearby.

3. Consider treatment options. When faced with a health decision, physicians give their treatment preference. However, *there is frequently more than one reasonable or viable alternative option, including the choice to do nothing.*

While all physicians have extensive education and training, they are not experts in everything—especially you. Aligning the immediate concerns with the best doctor type and experience with the issue can be difficult, but it is essential, especially if you are dealing with a serious health condition.

Try to understand why the physician recommended a particular treatment and do keep in mind the physician's experience level. Be sure to discuss the risks and benefits of the recommended treatment and alternatives. Then, go home and follow up with an internet search for quality information or information from other sources to support or challenge the recommendation. All the while, remember that the decisions about health are yours alone, not your doctor's.

> ## What to Do with Conflicting Health Information
>
> Health information is everywhere. Many of us can relate to hearing or reading news about preventing severe disease that conflicts with earlier news stories they heard. Even when we find relevant quality health information, can it be trusted as the one you should believe? It's often hard to tell when there are two or more quality sources of health information.
>
> Take eggs, for example. I recall when the public was told eggs were healthy, then they weren't, and then they were in moderation. I'm still unclear what the current stance on eggs is and who gets to make the rules about eggs being healthy. But the question to ask is, "Is this really true?" The answer to that will help you make your health decision.
>
> One method to evaluate information is to look for multiple quality websites that repeat the same information or get second opinions from health professionals. Don't be afraid to search for quality information that addresses the opposing perspective and then weigh the evidence for yourself before deciding what action to take.

Healthcare Guidelines as Health Information?

Few of us think about healthcare guidelines in context of health information, but they provide evidence-based recommendations for diagnosing, managing, and treating various health conditions and are foundational for informing both healthcare providers and patients about the best practices in medical care. These guidelines help standardize care, improve outcomes, and ensure that patients receive the most current and effective treatments based on the latest research.

Take diabetes, for example. The American Diabetes Association's (ADA's) *Standards of Medical Care in Diabetes* provides specific criteria for diagnosing diabetes.[2] Healthcare providers use these established guidelines to diagnose and manage the disease. If their patient falls within these guidelines, they'll recommend treatment. Criteria also can be found for prediabetes. If a doctor finds blood results that indicate prediabetes, they will talk about early intervention and management to prevent complications associated with the disease.

Healing vs. Remission: Reclaiming Our Power

In the medical world, the term "remission" is often used to describe conditions like cancer or Graves' disease that are no longer problematic or require medical attention. But remission can feel like a shadow hanging over us—a reminder that the disease might return, that true healing is out of reach. This perspective can rob us of hope and power.

But here's the truth: as people with incredible healing capacity, we have the right to say we're healed. Yes, if we slip back into unhealthy habits or fall into specific circumstances, there's a risk the condition could return—but that's a reality for everyone, not a life sentence. Healing is about more than just numbers on a chart; it's about taking ownership of our health and recognizing our ability to recover and thrive.

> We can't let the medical system define us. We must take control, acknowledge our healing, and live with the awareness that our choices matter. This isn't about ignoring risks—it's about embracing the power we have to heal and stay well. Healing is real, and it's within our reach.

Although healthcare guidelines are important and serve a valuable purpose of giving evidence to screen or treat disease, guidelines are also not perfect, and rarely do I hear anyone mention it. Few of us think about them at all, let alone question them. What should we know about healthcare guidelines to make better health decisions?

First, recognize that health guidelines are only a recommendation based on current available information. Guidelines are not strict rules to follow. Information and research used to make guidelines are limited and will never be all encompassing and include all the human factors at once, such as age, genetics, lifestyle, and preexisting conditions, along with any medications we may be taking. However, they are based on evidence, so they're worthy of consideration.

Second, not all guidelines are based on the highest quality of evidence. To explain this a little more, I want to give you a short lesson in quality of evidence which I think everyone should know. A cornerstone of classifying evidence in medicine is a hierarchical system called the Levels of Evidence (LOE), as shown in figure 4.2. LOE categorizes information into quality levels, from the lowest level VII, which is evidence from opinions of authorities and reports of expert committees, to the highest level I, which is evidence from a systematic review of all relevant randomized controlled trials (RCTs). RCT research is the gold standard and the best way to measure the effectiveness of screenings and treatments because they eliminate bias, such as selection bias, by removing investigators, participants, and data gatherers from knowing who is in the study group.

```
        Systemic
        Reviews
      Randomized
      Control Trials
      Cohort Studies
     Case Control Studies
   Case Series and Case Reports
   Editorials and Expert Opinion
```

Figure 4.2: Levels of Evidence

Why do I tell you this? Because not all healthcare guidelines are based on level I criteria. When few RCTs are available, guideline review experts must include other levels of evidence to help develop their decisions. But as a patient, we don't know this, so we trust all guidelines from our doctors and consider them equal.

Additionally, there is a chance of falling within guidelines and being treated when it isn't necessary. The book *Overdiagnosed, Making People Sick in Pursuit of Health* by Dr. H. Gilbert Welch, Dr. Lisa M. Schwartz, and Dr. Steven Woloshin, is a great study in challenging our traditional beliefs around getting regular checkups and the consequences of falling into a diagnosis and over-treating based on healthcare guidelines.

I guess what I'm trying to tell you is that you have options. Don't blindly trust and follow; be alert and aware. You get to decide what's best for you, not healthcare guidelines or otherwise.

Third, be aware that there may be multiple guidelines for one issue produced by different organizations, which can conflict. For example, I ran into this after having my knees replaced. There are conflicting guidelines about the use of antibiotics before dental procedures for patients with artificial joints. The American Academy of Orthopedic Surgeons

(AAOS) recommends antibiotics before dental cleaning procedures, whereas the American Dental Association (ADA) does not. This can confuse patients and healthcare providers about the best course of action. In these cases, weigh your options and make your best decision based on what you know.

Fourth, recognize that humans decide guidelines, each with their own biases and allegiances. Experts who make guideline decisions can include top specialists and physicians alongside medical consultants for pharmaceutical and medical device organizations. And again, when guideline decisions are made, it's not always in complete agreement with everyone on the panel of experts. If we could only learn about the dissenting opinions behind the guidelines, we could include that information in our decision-making. Regrettably, we will never know. So, we trust the guidelines because our doctors do, and they are our experts. Guidelines can also change overnight, as do the experts who make them and the doctors with their varying guidelines and opinions who use them.

Fifth, realize that people don't always fit neatly into the guidelines, because the guidelines are meant for *most* people, not *all* people. Guidelines throw us into one of two categories: normal or abnormal, but humans aren't all the same, all the time. Sometimes our medical numbers might indicate we're normal when we aren't, and abnormal when we're fine. Then, take into account borderline results. These are tricky because they may be erroneous or not problematic. It just depends on an individual's overall health, genetics, and circumstance. When screening results are borderline abnormal, we are at risk of being thrust into the category of a precondition, such as precancer, prediabetes, or prehypertension. What

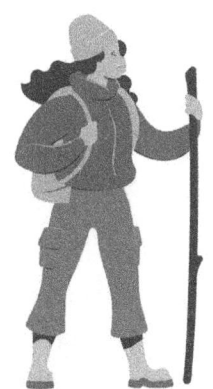

Guidelines can guide, but YOU rule!

happens next—treat or not treat—depends on the clinician's opinion and how you interpret the information and recommendation.

Like being a smart shopper when you're purchasing a car, I think it's good to be a smart healthcare consumer and think before you leap. You may not want to challenge the guidelines and defer to your healthcare provider, and that is your choice. But know that you may be susceptible to being thrust needlessly into a healthcare system. Balance the respected yet imperfect guidelines with your unique situation to help you make good-quality personalized health decisions.

Health Information from Our Social Circles

Multiple avenues of information influence our health decisions, but one of the most influential comes from those around us, friends, and family. We are more open to their persuasion because of our relationships.[3] Family, friends, and communities can support our decisions but can also exert pressures to conform, which can be positive or negative.

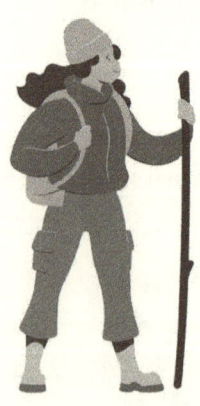

Stories may sway, but you get the final say.

How is it that our closest friends and family can persuade us so easily without statistical evidence to support their positions? They use powerful weapons of stories and testimonials, which are found to be more persuasive and influential on our decision-making than statistical evidence, especially where emotions are high. And when negative emotions run high, we are wired to be more responsive and receptive to information, which can have an even more potent effect on our decisions. Knowing we tend to be easily persuaded can help us put input from others into proper perspective.

Never Rely on a Single Source

Perhaps the most important takeaway from this chapter is that you should never rely on any single source of information as the basis for making a decision about your health. Don't trust only your own experiences. Websites can be faulty. Human beings (in the form of friends and physicians) can be biased. Even conclusions stated in a scientific paper could be outdated, replaced by later or additional research. As I've said many times, BE CURIOUS!

Good information leads to better health decisions. Where you get your information and what information you choose to believe can make the difference between healing quickly or not healing at all. Remember that you have control over what you choose to believe.

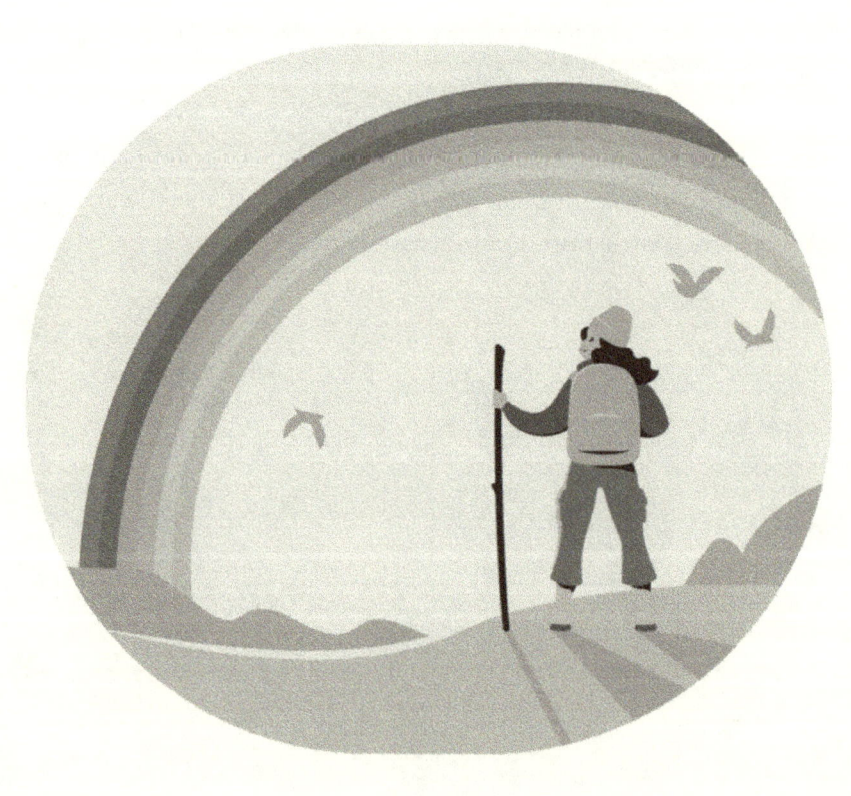

Part II

Developing Your Health Hero Superpowers

Now that you've gained a clear understanding of the forces working against your health in part I, you're better equipped to face them. But knowledge of these various forces against your health is only one piece of the puzzle. To truly make empowered and effective health decisions, you need to look inward at your unique approaches to health, and what will work best. In part II, we shift our focus from the outside world to the internal landscape. By developing a deeper understanding of yourself—your values, emotions, and how you make decisions—you can align your actions with what you truly need, and who you really are and want to be. This self-awareness will help you create a powerful health plan that is unique to only you. The key components are found in the following chapters:

- Defining your compass: a health philosophy for balance and harmony (chapter 5)
- Taking control of your decisions (chapter 6)
- Using decision-making tools (chapter 7)
- Developing confidence through attitude (chapter 8)
- Naming the unnamed: being able to articulate your emotions (chapter 9)

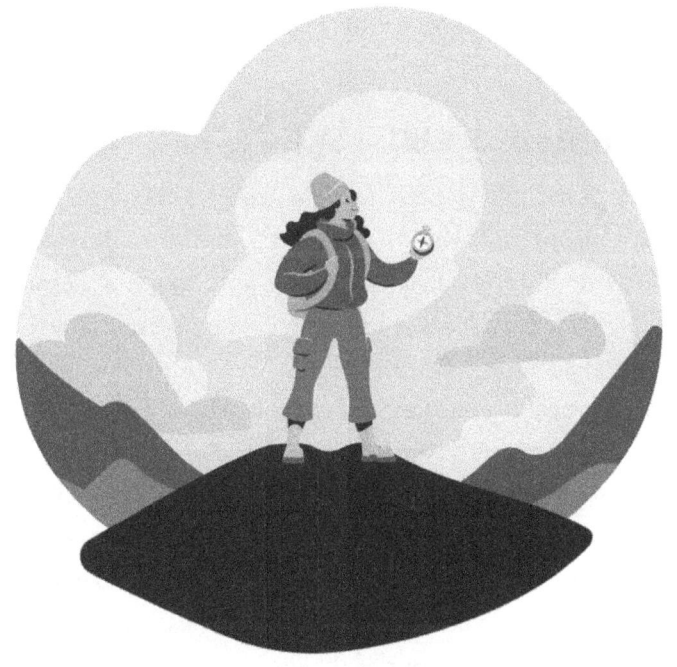

CHAPTER 5

Defining Your Compass: A Health Philosophy for Balance and Harmony

Most people limit the topic of health to the absence of disease or physical discomfort, but health is so much deeper than that. It's not just about how your body feels but also how your mind, spirit, and emotions intertwine. Achieving good health isn't just about reacting to symptoms or illnesses but about being aware of how you personally want to achieve balance and harmony with your health. I want to introduce you to the concept of a health philosophy. You already have one, but you likely haven't defined it. Once you do, you'll find that you can be much more efficient at making health decisions that help you heal faster and stay healthy.

What Is a Health Philosophy?

Your health philosophy represents your core beliefs and values about what health means and why it's important. It's the guiding vision that shapes your overall approach to well being. Your health philosophy is an invisible influence that drives your health decisions, especially those you make time and again.

When your health philosophy is clear, it acts as a compass, guiding your choices and actions toward what truly matters to you. For example, if your philosophy emphasizes natural healing approaches so you're not subject to medication side effects, you're more likely to seek out health interventions that include healthy lifestyle practices. This alignment creates harmony between your intentions and actions, making it easier to stay motivated and achieve your health goals.

When you don't choose actions that align with your health philosophy, several negative consequences can arise, each with its own impact. First, you may experience a feeling of disconnectedness and unsettledness. This is due to the cognitive dissonance you've created between what you value and what you are doing. For example, if your health philosophy values natural wellness, but you find yourself relying solely on pharmaceuticals without exploring lifestyle changes, this can lead to frustration and stress. The internal conflict between your beliefs and actions makes it hard to feel at peace with your health choices.

One common example of this that I've seen is when people who manage their health naturally decide nevertheless to take weight loss medications. Although they see positive weight loss results, they also lose muscle mass as a side effect. Losing muscle mass can result in a decrease of physical strength as well as a decreased overall basal metabolic rate, among other negative side effects. These side effects can have long-term consequences, such as having a lower metabolism once the medication is discontinued. Knowing this gives weight loss medication users a feeling of internal conflict—on one hand they want to lose weight, and on the other hand they don't want to compromise their health. The result is that they feel uneasy about being on the medication. Even though they are meeting their weight loss goals, they're not meeting the goals for their future health, so their actions aren't fully aligning with their health philosophy.

Another negative consequence that happens when a health philosophy doesn't align with health actions is that you will reduce your motivation to try or continue healthful practices. If you've compromised in one area of your health, why try to stay strong in all the other areas of health management? This can also lead you to experience lower satisfaction and overall well-being because you're not living in accordance with your true self. For example, if you believe in the importance of balanced living but constantly push yourself to the point of burnout, you're likely to feel unfulfilled and dissatisfied with your health status.

Now you can see how essential it is to align your health philosophy with your actions to avoid wasting time on interventions that don't "feel right." Let's align our health decisions and actions with our health philosophy so we can become who we want to be.

A Philosophy for the Future You

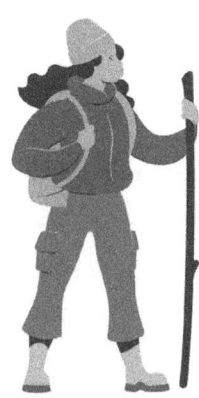

One easy way to map out your health philosophy is to envision your future self. What do you want your future health to look like? Knowing this will help you make health choices that help you become

When a health decision doesn't align with your health philosophy, you'll feel it—it just won't sit right.

your future healthy self. Even if you struggle with a current illness, you can still focus on the future healthy you and make health decisions based on that vision. Tell yourself, "Even though I don't feel good now, I will do what it takes to recover so that I can return back to my healthy self."

How you manage your health today probably hasn't been put in the context of how you want to see your health in ten years. So, I put some questions together to help you flesh out your health philosophy and what you envision for your health in the future. Use these questions to spark curiosity and embrace your answers—no one but you gets to define the vision for your future health. What you learn from these questions will help you form a philosophy and vision for what you want your health to be.

- **What do I want my future healthy self to look like?**
    - Reflect on what you want your health to be ten years from now.
- **What does "being healthy" mean to me?**
    - Reflect on your definition of health. Is it purely physical, or does it also include mental, emotional, and spiritual well-being? Understanding what health means to you can clarify your priorities and values.
- **What are my core beliefs about health and healing?**
    - Consider whether you believe in natural healing, the importance of medical interventions, or a balance between the two. Do you see health as something you actively cultivate, or do you believe it's largely out of your control?
- **How do I prioritize different aspects of my health?**
    - Think about which areas of health—such as nutrition, exercise, mental health, or social connections—are most important to you. This can help you identify where to focus your energy and resources.

- **What role do I believe prevention plays in maintaining health?**
  - Consider whether you prioritize preventive measures, like regular exercise and a healthy diet, or if you tend to focus more on addressing health issues as they arise.
- **How do I view the balance between traditional and alternative medicine?**
  - Reflect on your openness to alternative therapies like acupuncture, herbal medicine, or chiropractic care. Do you prefer a strictly conventional approach, or are you comfortable integrating different types of interventions?
- **What are my beliefs about the mind-body connection?**
  - Explore your thoughts on how mental and emotional health impacts physical health. Do you believe stress and emotions play a significant role in physical well-being?
- **What past experiences have shaped my views on health?**
  - Consider how your personal history, such as past illnesses, family health traditions, or experiences with healthcare providers, has influenced your health philosophy.
- **How do my cultural, spiritual, or religious beliefs influence my approach to health?**
  - Reflect on whether and how your cultural or spiritual background shapes your views on health, healing, and the body.
- **What are my long-term health goals?**
  - Think about what you hope to achieve in the future regarding your health. How do these goals align with your broader life philosophy and values?

- **How do I balance short-term comfort with long-term health benefits?**
  - Consider how you approach decisions involving trade-offs, like choosing between immediate comfort (e.g., indulging in unhealthy food) and long-term health benefits (e.g., maintaining a healthy diet). This question addresses present bias, mentioned in chapter 2.

A health philosophy doesn't have to be overly detailed to be effective; it just needs to be clear enough to guide your health decisions consistently. Here's how you can bring your answers together to form a general health philosophy:

1. **Identify common themes.** As you answer each question, look for recurring themes or patterns. For example, if you find that many of your answers emphasize natural healing, prevention, and the importance of mental health, these themes are central to your philosophy.

2. **Distill key beliefs.** Boil down these themes into a few core beliefs. For example, you might realize that your health philosophy centers around the belief that health is a holistic balance of physical, mental, and emotional well-being, and that prevention is key to maintaining this balance.

3. **Create a guiding statement.** Formulate a simple guiding statement that captures your core beliefs. For instance, "I believe in maintaining health through holistic, preventive measures that nurture both the body and mind." This statement doesn't have to cover every detail but should encapsulate your most important beliefs.

4. **Stay flexible.** Your health philosophy should be flexible enough to adapt to new experiences and information. It's not set in stone but serves as a general guide that can evolve over time as you learn more about yourself and what works for you.

5. **Apply it consistently.** Once you've distilled your philosophy, use it as a touchstone for making health decisions. Whenever you're faced with a choice—whether it's about diet, exercise, or medical treatment—refer back to your guiding statement to ensure your actions align with your core beliefs.

Health philosophies can vary widely based on individual values, beliefs, and approaches to well-being. Here is a sampling of different philosophies I've seen people adopt:

- A **holistic** health philosophy emphasizes the balance of physical, emotional, mental, and spiritual well-being, with a focus on natural remedies, preventive care, and practices like meditation, yoga, and complementary therapies.
- A **preventive** health philosophy prioritizes proactive measures to prevent illness before it starts, such as regular checkups, vaccinations, and maintaining a healthy lifestyle based on scientific research.
- A **minimalist** health philosophy advocates for simplicity, trusting in the body's natural ability to heal and avoiding overreliance on medical interventions unless absolutely necessary.
- An **evidence-based** health philosophy is grounded in scientific research, with a focus on medical treatments and lifestyle changes that have been proven effective through rigorous studies.
- A **spiritual** health philosophy connects health to spiritual beliefs and practices, incorporating prayer, meditation, and other rituals, with a strong emphasis on faith and spiritual healing.
- An **integrative** health philosophy combines conventional medical treatments with complementary therapies, seeking to balance the strengths of both modern medicine and alternative practices.

Each of these philosophies reflects a different perspective on health and healing, and individuals may choose one or blend elements from several to create a personalized approach that aligns with their unique values and goals.

From Philosophy to Action

Having a philosophy is one thing. Using it to propel your health forward is another. In part III of this book, I cover in more depth the elements that will help you take actions consistent with your philosophy, but here is a quick preview so you can see how the components fit together.

1. Your **health philosophy** is the destination you aim to reach—a state of optimal health according to your values and beliefs. A health philosophy is visionary in that it sets the overarching beliefs and ideals that guide your understanding of health.

2. **Health approach** is the mode of transportation or the general route you choose to get there—whether it's through holistic practices, lifestyle approaches, conventional medicine, or a blend of all three. It outlines the general strategies and methodologies you will adopt under your health philosophy. (See chapter 11.)

3. **A health plan** is the itinerary for the journey—specific, actionable steps, goals, and timelines that keep you on track and ensure you're making progress toward your destination. It's the actionable road map that guides your day-to-day efforts toward achieving your health objectives. I walk you through how to develop a health plan in chapter 16.

4. **Health goals** are the actionable steps in the health plan, with timelines. They provide the data that determines if each of the steps you choose are helpful in achieving your target. There are often many goals that fall under the health plan that translate into daily and weekly action. This component is also covered in chapter 16.

In sum, a health philosophy is **visionary**, a health approach is **strategic**, a health plan is **actionable**, and health goals are **targeted**. By thoughtfully aligning your health goals with your philosophy, approach, and plan, you now have a practical and motivating path toward the well-being you aspire to achieve.

Example of Implementing the Health Philosophy Approach

As a more concrete example of how these four components can drive better health and healthcare decisions, let's look at Roberta, who was just diagnosed with Epstein-Barr virus, or EBV, and she's trying to navigate her way toward better health. Here's how she might articulate her health philosophy, approach, and plan, followed by setting specific health goals.

- Roberta's health philosophy centers around a belief in holistic wellness. She recognizes that true health is not just about eliminating symptoms but achieving balance across her physical, mental, and emotional well-being. She understands that her body has an incredible ability to heal itself, and she is committed to supporting that natural process by nurturing all aspects of her health.

- Based on her philosophy, Roberta's health approach could involve combining conventional medicine with natural and lifestyle-based interventions. To manage the effects of EBV, she decides to focus on strengthening her immune system, managing stress, and maintaining a balanced diet. She plans to work closely with her conventional healthcare providers to monitor her condition while incorporating complementary therapies like herbal supplements, meditation, and regular physical activity.

- Because she is committed to holistic wellness and wants an approach that combines conventional and complementary practices, Roberta develops a health plan that describes specific actionable steps that she can integrate into her daily life, such as following a diet rich in anti-inflammatory foods, meeting with a certified herbalist and incorporating herbal therapies to recover from EBV, practicing healing meditation daily to support Roberta's belief in healing, and ensuring she gets enough rest to support her immune system. She also schedules regular checkups with her healthcare provider.

- The actionable steps created in Roberta's health plan become her immediate health goals that she can convert into a checklist of actions she wants to complete in the next six weeks. Items on her list include meeting with her healthcare provider in six weeks, incorporating three anti-inflammatory foods into her diet daily for six weeks, meeting with an herbalist once next week and taking weekly herbs for the following five weeks, meditating every day for fifteen minutes, and sleeping eight hours every night.

By following this structured approach, Roberta has given herself the best chance to manage her condition effectively. Her holistic approach helps her address not just the physical symptoms of EBV but also the mental and emotional aspects, leading to better symptom management and overall well-being. By taking control of her health in this way, Roberta is more likely to experience an improvement in her condition. It can do the same for you.

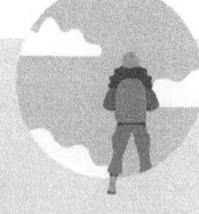

Q&A WITH ALICE: DOES THIS NEED TO BE SO COMPLICATED?

Thinking about a health philosophy and approach, plan, and goals feels overwhelming. So I'm not surprised when people say to me, "Can't you simplify the process so I can improve my health more quickly?"

I get it—this attitude is why most Americans choose quick, fast approaches, like just taking a quick pill. But when we do that, we miss out on potential healing and learning opportunities.

Taking care of our health requires a level of strategy that past generations never had to consider. Back in the day, our foods were naturally more nutritious, physical activity was woven into the fabric of daily life, and doctors didn't have the option to overprescribe—because those options simply didn't exist. Fast-forward to today, and we find ourselves navigating a highly complex health landscape, where processed foods dominate, sedentary lifestyles are the norm, and the healthcare system often prioritizes quick fixes over true wellness. This environment demands that we think critically about our health choices. We can no longer afford to be passive recipients of whatever the system offers; instead, we must be proactive, informed, and strategic in our approach to health. It's about reclaiming our power and making decisions that truly serve our best interests, rather than becoming victims of a system that isn't always aligned with our well-being.

Consider Your Impact on Others

No philosophy of health can be complete unless it takes into account what I call "health liability"—meaning the impact that your state of health has on those around you. Every decision or action we take can have ripple effects, not just on our personal health but potentially on others around us. Each health decision contributes to a larger ecosystem of health and well-being. It's a reminder of the significant impact our personal choices have, not just on ourselves but also on the broader community.

Consider when we poorly manage our health. This behavior leads to chronic diseases, reduces our quality of life, and costs us lots of money on healthcare. But if too many of us poorly manage our health, the consequences extend beyond just us; they affect the healthcare system and society as a whole. This, in fact, is what we're seeing today. Our healthcare system is overloaded with diseases that could have been prevented by living healthier. Our healthcare costs are also higher because of our poor health choices.

Take it back to a personal level. Let's say we choose unhealthy fast food over vegetables and fruits purchased at our local grocery store, and everyone around us does the same. What happens next? The demand for fast food goes up and more fast food restaurants appear, and access to healthy foods go down—the grocery store starts to reduce how many healthy foods they carry.

Addressing health liability is not about assigning blame but rather about encouraging a sense of responsibility and awareness. By understanding that our health choices have broader implications, we can make more meaningful health decisions—they matter not just to us, but to those around us. My hope is that this awareness will lead us all to take more personal responsibility for our health decisions.

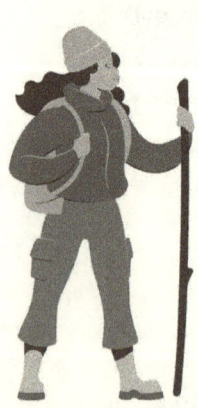

Everything we do with our health has a collective impact on others. Let it be a positive one.

While discussing health liability might be uncomfortable, I believe it's absolutely necessary. While we have the freedom to make our own health choices (of which I am thankful), we must also recognize that we are responsible for the consequences of those choices. Simply considering how our health choices impact others will hopefully promote better understanding of how what we do impacts those around us.

A better understanding of health liability can shape your health philosophy much like how the environmental movement promoted recycling. Just as recycling efforts evolved based on the significant impact that individual actions collectively can have on the environment, recognizing the broader consequences of your health-related choices can deepen your appreciation for how these actions affect not only your own health but also the well-being of those around you. I hope this awareness inspires you to adopt a more comprehensive health philosophy that considers both personal benefits and the collective impact.

As with the recycling movement, individual responsibility can lead to widespread change. Every decision to recycle a bottle, like every decision to choose a healthier lifestyle, contributes to a larger effort that benefits everyone. This shift in perspective can encourage you to prioritize preventive care, healthful behaviors, and a health approach that values us all. As you integrate this perspective into your health philosophy, you may find yourself more committed to making thoughtful and purposeful decisions. Just as recycling has become a simple yet powerful tool for environmental conservation, thoughtful health decisions can be a potent means of improving our health and health culture. I hope you consider it as you create your health philosophy and approach.

Creating a Solid Foundation

Few good things in life come without some effort. If you want to heal, it will take focused attention and discipline to speed up the healing

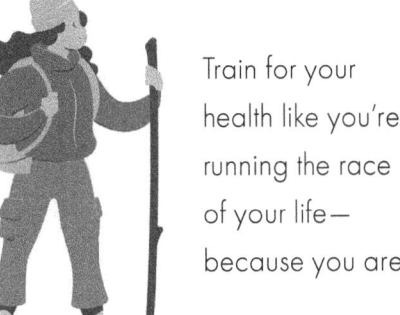

Train for your health like you're running the race of your life — because you are!

and recovery process. I know that may not be what people want to hear, but the truth is, we need to approach healing like an athlete, with undivided, focused attention, with the goal of healing in mind. That is what the recommended steps I outline in this book will help you do. Being clear about your basic health philosophy will provide a stable foundation that will help you sort through the many options and decisions you'll face, no matter whether your goal is continued health, improved fitness, or resolving a health concern.

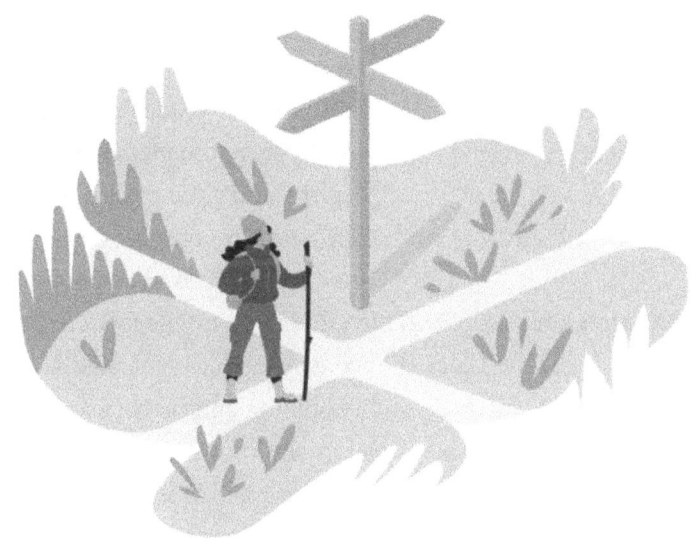

CHAPTER 6

Taking Control of Your Decisions

Why is it that two people in the same health scenario facing the same health decision come to completely different conclusions? Or why do some people handle health decisions with ease, while others struggle? Or why do some people diligently manage their health, while others don't? It might be circumstance, but it's more likely that it's our individual temperament that is responsible for these differences. Personality drives behavior. It's impossible to change our inherent traits. The best we can do is recognize and understand our individual temperament and personality so we can recognize when and how it is helping us stay healthy, and when it gets in the way.

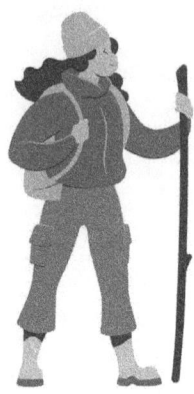

Personality drives behavior.

Meet Tanya, well known for being an overthinker. Tanya is the type of person who can turn even the simplest health decision into a full-blown research project. When she wakes up with a slight headache, most people would grab some water or maybe an aspirin and take a nap. Not Tanya. She starts by consulting five different medical websites, reading articles on hydration, stress, and sleep, and then dives into online forums for headache sufferers. Two hours later, she's convinced she might need a complete overhaul of her diet, a new ergonomic pillow, and perhaps a meditation retreat to address her stress levels. Before she knows it, she's overwhelmed and paralyzed by all the information—and her headache is still there, now accompanied by a newfound tension in her shoulders.

On the flip side, meet Mike, the "It'll be fine" guy. Mike's the kind of person who shrugs off health concerns like they're just a passing breeze. When his knee starts acting up, does he slow down or consult a doctor? Nope. He decides to power through his morning run, convinced it's just a fluke. Fast-forward a week, and Mike's hobbling around, refusing to admit that his knee might need some rest—or, heaven forbid, actual medical attention. But hey, in Mike's world, everything eventually "works itself out," even if he's limping his way through it.

Tanya and Mike couldn't be more different, yet both of them show how personality can get in the way of making good health decisions. Tanya's overthinking makes her hesitate, while Mike's underthinking leads him to ignore potential issues. The truth is, most of us fall somewhere in between Tanya and Mike, and recognizing these tendencies can help us strike a better balance. So as you explore your own personality, remember: a little self-awareness can go a long way toward getting out of your own way.

How Does Your Personality Impact Your Health?

Personality is the unique blend of traits, habits, and tendencies that shape how we see the world—and how we respond to it, including when it comes to our health. Whether we realize it or not, everything we do is influenced by our personality, from the smallest choices to the biggest decisions. That's why, before you make your next health decision, it's essential to uncover your personality type. Understanding your own tendencies can reveal why you do what you do and help you navigate your health journey with greater self-awareness.

Just like our DNA, our personality is uniquely ours. It guides us in making decisions—whether we approach things with caution, dive in headfirst, or take the scenic route. The way we care for ourselves often reflects these distinct traits. While our personality can sometimes propel us toward great health choices, it can also trip us up or slow down our healing. By recognizing these patterns, we can learn to harness the best of our traits and sidestep the pitfalls.

Psychologists have been studying this very thing for years, and they've found that understanding our personality traits can significantly impact our health outcomes.[1] By becoming aware of our natural tendencies, we can harness our strengths and counterbalance our weaknesses, making more intentional and effective health decisions. The better we understand ourselves, the more clearly we can see what needs to be done to get us healthy again.

Now, it's time to uncover your unique personality type. Below, I give you six choices to go through; you must choose one trait out of each. The traits are summarized in table 6.1; fuller descriptions follow.

Personality Dimension	Strengths	Challenges
Proactive	Actively prevents issues; reduces illness risk	Can overdo interventions, leading to wasted effort
Reactive	Quickly addresses issues as they arise	May miss early signs of preventable conditions
Analytical	Thorough decision-making based on data	Overanalyzes, leading to indecision
Intuitive	Relies on self-awareness and instinct	May overlook critical facts in favor of gut feelings
Cautious	Minimizes risks; follows proven methods	Avoids risks, potentially missing beneficial treatments
Risk-taking	Open to new solutions and ideas	Engages in risky practices; may ignore professional advice
Social	Seeks support; values opinions of others	Easily influenced by others, even when harmful
Independent	Tailors health management to personal preferences	May miss valuable support or perspectives from others
Optimistic	Maintains positivity and control over health	Underestimates risks, delaying care
Pessimistic	Vigilant; seeks prompt medical care	Excessive worry; may avoid care or options
Structured	Consistent with routines and plans	Struggles with adapting to new health plans
Flexible	Adapts easily to changing circumstances	Inconsistent in maintaining health routines

Table 6.1: Summary of Personality Attributes

As you read through the following list, remember that there's no right or wrong type, and no one personality is better than another—you'll discover there are pros and cons to them all. In fact, at times we will shift between different categories, depending on the situation. There are also varying degrees within each type—none of us are all or nothing. Still, we each have a dominant personality that tends to guide our health behaviors. Don't worry if you don't fit perfectly into one category; just pick the one that matches you the most closely.

1. Proactive vs. Reactive

- **Proactive:** If you're proactive, you actively manage your health by taking preventive measures like scheduling regular checkups and maintaining a healthy lifestyle. This approach can significantly reduce your risk of illness, as many potential issues can be prevented. However, being too proactive might lead to unnecessary efforts, such as seeking interventions for conditions that are rare or at least that are unlikely to be affecting you. This can result in wasted time, money, and resources on treatments or preventive measures that aren't truly needed for maintaining optimal health.
- **Reactive:** Reactive individuals address health issues quickly as they arise. This means that they will not let conditions fester for long. However, being reactive can lead to overreliance and utilization of medical interventions and less utilization of lifestyle and complementary interventions (which I discuss in part III). This approach might delay an early diagnosis and subsequent treatment of preventable conditions.

2. Analytical vs. Intuitive

- **Analytical:** Analytical individuals manage health using detailed information, diving into data, and exploring various options when it comes to their health. Although this thorough approach seems beneficial when managing health, it also leads to chasing health management approaches that aren't necessarily helpful or needed. It also might lead to overanalyzing ("paralysis by analysis"), which could delay action.

- **Intuitive:** If you're intuitive, you rely on gut feelings and heartfelt emotions to drive health behaviors. Take exercise, for example. An intuitive person would exercise because their gut instinct tells them to—their bodies are speaking. Intuitive personalities have a higher self-awareness and so have a sense of what to do when managing their health. However, they also may miss or overlook critical information and signs that aren't intuitive. Back to the exercise example, maybe exercise isn't a good idea, because they have an undiagnosed heart condition. Intuitives are at risk of missing the facts because the feelings dominate.

3. Cautious vs. Risk-Taking

- **Cautious:** Cautious personalities tend to be risk-averse, so they follow established medical guidance and advice and avoid risky behaviors. Although this minimizes some dangers, it also might lead them to miss the counter-perspective and so creates a one-sided viewpoint. A cautious person may also avoid beneficial treatments due to perceived risks.

- **Risk-taking:** Risk-takers are open to out-of-the-box ways to manage their health. You'll find them exploring alternative treatments and new health trends, which may help them discover effective solutions others overlook. However, they may also engage in unsafe health practices or disregard professional advice.

4. Social vs. Independent

- **Social:** If you're social, you value social support and seek advice from family and friends and are more likely to seek others' opinions. The flip side is that you also are more likely to be swayed to participate or partake in health management practices that could potentially compromise your health. For example, let's say your coworkers are all using a daily protein shake for six weeks to lose weight. Because you are social and want to lose weight, you decide it would be a good idea to join your coworkers. During that time, you see your doctor and find that protein shakes aren't good for you, because of a kidney condition. The social aspect tipped your decisions to participate to the point that you didn't consider the risks it might have on your kidney condition.
- **Independent:** Independent folks prefer to manage their health on their own. If that's you, you may base your health management on personal research. This autonomy gives you a tailored health management approach, but beware that it may also cause you to miss out on valuable perspectives or support from others.

5. Optimistic vs. Pessimistic

- **Optimistic:** If you're an optimist, you maintain a positive outlook on your health in general. Optimists generally feel like they have control over their well-being. However, you might underestimate health risks because of your positivity, potentially delaying care.
- **Pessimistic:** With a more cautious or negative outlook, you may be vigilant about health and seek prompt medical attention. This vigilance can sometimes lead to unnecessary stress or avoidance of necessary care. It may also impede the full capacity of healing because of worry and disbelief that healing is possible. It can also make you a skeptic, which can be healthy if kept in check. But it can

also narrow your options to fully manage your health. For example, a pessimist might not believe doctors can help them much and seek their care less frequently.

6. Structured vs. Flexible

- **Structured:** If you are structured, you thrive on routines and schedules, ensuring consistent health maintenance and adherence to treatment plans. Additionally, if a new routine is required and you're confident about it, you will easily adapt to it. However, you might struggle with adapting to new health management plans if it throws off your routine or structured way of thinking.

- **Flexible:** If you are flexible, you are adaptable and can adjust your health strategies based on changing circumstances. While this responsiveness is beneficial, it may sometimes lead to a lack of consistency in maintaining regular health practices. Or you may want to continue to try new health management tactics when they're not helpful or needed because you're so open that anything goes.

What Does It All Mean?

So which personality types were you? If you're looking at a hard copy of this book, circle your answers in table 6.2; if reading an electronic version highlight the terms you chose or make a separate list of your choices.

WHAT DOMINANT PERSONALITY TYPES AM I: THIS OR THAT?	
Proactive	Reactive
Analytical	Intuitive
Cautious	Risk-Taking
Social	Independent
Optimistic	Pessimistic
Structured	Flexible

Table 6.2: What Are Your Dominant Personality Types?

Now that you've identified the personality traits that resonate with you, congratulations—you've just discovered your unique health persona! Think of it as your personal health identity, a blend of traits that guide how you navigate your health journey. Whether you're a proactive analyst or a flexible optimist, understanding your health persona helps you recognize your strengths and potential blind spots when it comes to making health decisions.

Why does this matter? Because knowing yourself is the

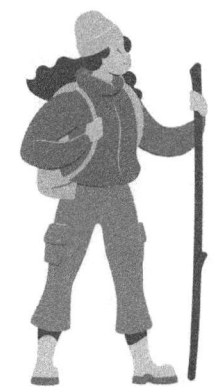

To make better health decisions, we must first understand ourselves—because sometimes the biggest obstacle to our well-being is the person in the mirror.

first step to managing your health in a way that works for you. If you're a proactive type, you're likely someone who takes charge of your health before issues arise, making you great at prevention. But if you're more reactive, you might find that you respond well to challenges, making you resilient when it counts. Similarly, analytical thinkers excel at researching and making data-driven decisions, while intuitive types might trust their gut to guide them. Whether you're cautious or risk-taking, social or independent, optimistic or pessimistic, structured or flexible, each trait brings something valuable to the table. Yet the exact opposite can be true. The negative traits can collide, creating an unhelpful mix of traits that slows down your healing or health-seeking progress.

So, the next time you're faced with a health decision, think about your health persona and how it can guide you. Lean into your strengths, be aware of your tendencies, and remember that understanding yourself is the key to creating a health strategy that helps you be healthier faster.

How is your personality influencing you?

Remember that there is no "perfect" temperament. The purpose of reviewing these aspects of personality is to help you course-correct if one personality trait is dominating how you manage your health to your detriment. Having reviewed the descriptions, can you start to see how your personality traits impact how you manage your health? Your personality takes you down one path of health navigation. But could you be able to see the forks in the road that could take you down a better path?

Personality and Critical Decisions

The personality traits just covered will affect the way you manage your health, and that's a fact. Nowhere is that more visible than when you face important health decisions, or even when you manage a common health challenge, like losing weight. Let me illustrate how much personality can impact our health choices and actions.

Terri was a client of mine years ago. She realized she needed to lose weight, and she was willing to do anything—a dream client, you might think. Her open-minded and accommodating nature made her a pleasure to work with. She readily embraced new exercise routines and successfully transformed several negative lifestyle habits into positive ones.

While her personality traits appeared predominantly positive, Terri's open nature rendered her susceptible to the influence of her friends, particularly in matters concerning diets and supplements. Terri ended up spending significant sums each month on supplements that offered minimal benefit, not to mention profited her friends. With her open-minded tendencies, Terri found herself engaging in and abandoning five different diets during our work together. Our agreed-upon approach often veered off track the very next day.

Terri wasn't the first client that had the tendency to shift their health strategy from one moment to the next. We all are tempted to get off track at times, but Terri and clients like her are so easily persuaded to try new interventions (hello bandwagon effect!), it becomes nearly impossible to coach them.

What was causing Terri to be so easily persuaded? It was her personality. The very one that was positive in many aspects was also keeping her from achieving her desired outcome—weight loss. This doesn't have to happen to you. Personality plays a very important role in our decision-making. Now that you've discovered your unique health persona, you're already one step closer to understanding how you navigate your health journey. But there's more to the picture—your decision-making personality plays a crucial role in how you choose the best path forward. Just like your health persona guides your approach, your decision-making style determines how you evaluate options and make choices. Let's dive deeper into how you tend to make health decisions.

The Four Styles of Decision-Making

We all have our unique approach to making health decisions. Some of us dive in and decide quickly, while others prefer to gather all the information before making a move. Understanding your decision-making style can be a game changer. When you recognize your tendencies, you can play to your strengths and counterbalance any less helpful habits. By doing so, you'll make smarter choices not just for yourself, but for those you care about as well.[2]

There are four tendencies: conceptual, behavioral, analytical, and directive.

1. I call them C-BAD because it helps you see the bad in your health decision-making. Read through each one and pick the one that resonates with the way you typically make health decisions. I recommend you read through them all before landing on a predominant type. I'm sure you'll notice that it's easy to discover the type of those who are closest to you. So, if you're not sure which of the four styles you are, ask someone close to you what they think.

Conceptual Decision-Makers

Conceptual decision-makers think outside of the box when it comes to managing their health. They are willing to try unconventional approaches to address their health concerns, often with seemingly unlimited patience. Conceptuals are comfortable with uncertainty to some extent and are willing to take more risk to heal by trying strategies out of the normal approaches. These individuals have a set vision of what they want their health to be, although they are not so clear about the goals to get them there.

Let's say you went to the doctor with shoulder pain, and they told you that you needed shoulder surgery. As a conceptual decision-maker faced with what to do next, you might initially be reluctant to have surgery.

Instead, you'd prefer exploring alternative methods and complementary therapies such as deep tissue massages with cupping, ice and heat treatments, and acupuncture. Only after exhausting enough other options in a reasonable time frame would you consider surgery.

If you resonate with this style, here are some ways to maximize your conceptual strengths while staying mindful of the potential pitfalls:

1. Diligently research new interventions to avoid wasting time, money, or risking your health on unproven methods.
2. Base your health decisions on facts and consider the probabilities associated with diagnoses and treatment options. For example, what would the risk be if you wait to get shoulder surgery?
3. Incorporate a balanced approach by combining medical, complementary, and lifestyle strategies, rather than over-relying on a single method.
4. Gather insights from individuals who embrace a different one of the three decision-making styles to guarantee a more comprehensive choice.

Conceptual insight: Conceptual decision-makers excel in situations where traditional options fall short, like when medical interventions only treat a disease, but not reverse it. A conceptual's innovative thinking often leads to remarkable ideas and suggestions of other approaches to try that other people might not have considered otherwise.

Behavioral Decision-Makers

Behavioral decision-makers, unknowingly most of the time, prioritize their emotions and the feelings of others when navigating choices. Their decision-making process is driven from the heart, not necessarily the head (evidence). Many times, you'll hear behavioral decision-makers say statements like, "I feel like I should..." or "This feels like the best option."

As a behavioral decision-maker, how would you approach the shoulder surgery dilemma? You might tend to heavily weigh the recommendations of your close friends and family. You'd also be inclined to place significant trust in your doctor's judgment, often without exploring alternative options. While you might seek information online, the most influential factor would be the opinions of the people in your life, and how their advice makes you feel, regardless of the facts.

If the behavioral decision-making style resonates with you, here are ways to harness your behavioral strengths while staying mindful of potential drawbacks:

1. Acknowledge that the emotions you experience are momentary. Don't let emotions dominate the decision. Instead, allocate a specific time, like 24 hours, for these feelings to subside before making a health decision.
2. Seek input from trusted friends and family who possess a directive, analytical, or conceptual decision-making style, especially for significant health decisions.
3. Invest extra time and effort in verifying the facts and ensuring that the information you're receiving is accurate.

Behavioral insight: Behavioral decision-makers are genuine, empathetic, and emotionally attuned, so they are wonderful providers of hope and comfort during times of health challenges that are not their own. They also can be inconsistent and fickle when it comes to making health decisions. So, if you are a behavioral, make sure that you recognize when your feelings are dominating your actions. If they are, take a deep breath and ask yourself what the facts are, and stick with those to help you make a health decision.

Analytical Decision-Makers

Analytical decision-makers are the epitome of thoroughness and detail when it comes to making health choices. They fearlessly dive into oceans of data, especially in the face of ambiguity or uncertainty, although many times it's at the expense of time spent.

If you had an analytical decision-making style, you'd meticulously trace the shoulder pain's origins, scour the internet for information, consult friends and colleagues who've encountered similar issues, and engage in extensive contemplation before reaching a conclusion about what to do about it.

If the analytical decision-making style strikes a chord with you, consider these strategies to amplify your analytical strengths while keeping potential pitfalls in check:

1. Allow your emotional side some time to catch up with your logical assessment. Dedicate a few moments to gauge your emotional response to the situation.
2. Impose time constraints on your decision-making process to avert analysis paralysis.
3. Compile the most pertinent and promising information and options, ranking them with the most favorable choice at the top. Limit your options to three to five.
4. Establish a decision threshold for when "good enough" is truly sufficient.
5. Seek input from individuals possessing one of the other three decision-making styles to ensure a well-rounded choice.

Analytical insight: Analytical decision-makers excel at offering sound advice to others because of their meticulous and informed recommendations. They will even do all the legwork to find the necessary information to make a good health decision for someone else.

Directive Decision-Makers

Directive decision-makers favor swift and unwavering choices, harboring a subtle disdain for uncertainty and ambiguity. They rely on cold, hard facts and the counsel of trustworthy sources to steer their healthcare decisions. They need good information to make their health decisions, but not too much because they aren't interested in deliberating on next steps more than necessary.

If you had a directive decision-making style and were faced with the shoulder surgery scenario, you wouldn't dwell on the next course of action for long. Your choice would be heavily influenced by the initial information you encounter. If the doctor recommends surgery and this sounded reasonable, you'd promptly schedule the procedure for the following week. Alternatively, you might find two or three options and weigh them out, all the while reasoning that the sooner you decide, the sooner you'll return to your normal life, pain-free.

If the directive decision-making style aligns with your tendencies, consider these strategies to maximize your directive strengths while maintaining a balanced approach:

1. Explore two or three significantly different alternatives from what you've initially found, then assess if your inclination remains unchanged.

2. Seek input from a trusted confidant to gauge if your haste is justified.

3. Delve into the broader implications of rushing your decision, weighing what you stand to gain against potential losses. Is expediting truly essential? What might you miss by not taking the time for a more comprehensive exploration of options?

4. Take a moment to scrutinize the facts to differentiate objective truths from subjective opinions.

5. Dedicate a little time to consider your emotional response to the chosen approach, ensuring your feelings play a role in the decision-making process.

Directive insight: Directive decision-makers are exceptionally logical, often acting as the voice of reason when others grapple with overwhelming decisions. You also excel in providing validation for seemingly rational options and devising quick solutions. Need someone to give you a solid, quick health decision? Ask a directive!

Now that you've explored both your health persona and decision-making tendency, you're equipped with powerful insights into how you approach your well-being. But understanding these aspects of yourself is only the beginning. The real magic happens when you bring it all together by aligning your personality and decision-making style to create a cohesive and confident health strategy.

The Power of Knowing Yourself: Making Better Health Decisions

Now you know why two different people who have similar health decisions to make come to two completely different decisions. You have in your hands both your health persona and your decision-making tendency—two key pieces of the puzzle that shape how you navigate your well-being. We are unique, yet we all have similar types of tendencies that we work within. Understanding your personality gives you a clear picture of your strengths and natural inclinations, while recognizing your decision-making tendency helps you identify your innate tendency to make health choices. Together, these insights form a powerful foundation for making health decisions that are not only aligned with who you are but are also balanced and thoughtful. Health decisions aren't black and white anymore, they're the color of you.

Why does this matter? When you combine the self-awareness of your health persona with the awareness of your decision-making tendencies, you're better equipped to avoid pitfalls, embrace your strengths, and ultimately make decisions that lead to better outcomes. It's like having a personalized guide to help you think outside of yourself and make better health decisions when you're not thinking your clearest. But you don't need a guide, because you can now warn yourself.

So, as you move forward, keep these insights about yourself close. Go back to them often and make sure you're understanding the parts they play in your health decisions. This will help you navigate the complex landscape of health decisions with confidence, clarity, and a deeper understanding of yourself. After all, when you know yourself, you can take control of your health and steer it in the direction you want to go.

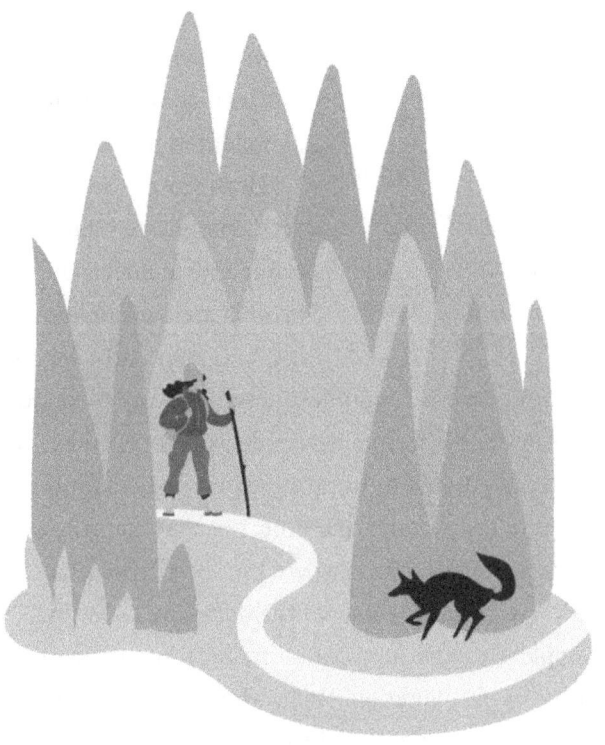

CHAPTER 7

From Personality to Reality: Using Decision-Making Tools

Understanding your personality and decision-making tendencies is the first step in recognizing how you naturally approach health decisions. But when it's time to move beyond tendencies and into the realm of reality, decision-making tools become your anchor. These tools help you balance your personality-driven instincts with clear, objective reasoning, ensuring that your choices aren't just guided by who

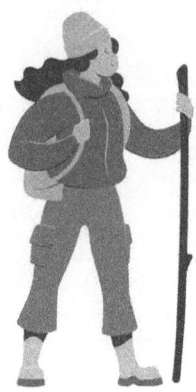

When personality leads us astray, decision-making tools can save the day.

you are, but by what's truly best for your health. Now that you know yourself better, let's explore the tools that can guide you to make more confident, informed decisions.

Healthcare decisions can be very complicated. Surprisingly, even though we use decision-making tools in other areas of our lives—like choosing a career path, buying a home, or even deciding on a vacation destination—many of us don't think to apply these same tools to our health decisions. Yet these tools can be just as valuable in guiding us toward the best choices for our well-being. We don't need to use them all the time, but they can be especially helpful when we're facing decisions where the "best" choice isn't obvious, or when we know our innate personality might lead us astray.

For example, imagine someone deciding whether or not to undergo surgery for a chronic condition. Dani, who used a decision-making tool, carefully weighed the benefits and risks of surgery against other options, like physical therapy or medication. By using the tool, she realized that surgery might be more invasive than necessary and opted for a less risky approach that still aligned with her goals. On the other hand, Melissa, who didn't use a tool, quickly decided to go through with the surgery without fully considering alternative treatments, only to face complications that might have been avoided with more thorough decision-making. Tools like these can save us from making hasty decisions that we might regret later.

So, how do you know when a tool might be helpful? If you're facing a choice that feels overwhelming, or if you've been burned by a poor decision in the past, it's a good sign that a decision-making tool could be your best friend. These tools help you sort through your options, prioritize what matters most, and ultimately make a more confident, informed choice.[1]

Five Tools for Improved Decision-Making

Here are my five favorite decision-making tools, ranging from the simplest to the most complex. Each one has its own strengths, and knowing when to use them can make all the difference in your health decisions:

1. **Pros and Cons List:** Think of this as the quick and dirty tool for decision-making. When you're in a hurry and need to make a choice, simply jot down the factors in favor of one option and those against it (see figure 7.1). This method shines in situations where you need a fast decision, and the upsides and downsides are easy to spot. It's perfect for those times when you just need a little clarity to move forward.

Is This Health Intervention Right For Me?
Pros and Cons

Pros ↓	Cons ↓

Figure 7.1: Pros and Cons List

2. **Plan-Do-Check-Act (PDCA) Cycle:** If you like to test the waters before diving in, or you want to keep things simple and clear, this

is a simple method. PDCA, which stands for Plan-Do-Check-Act, is a well-known approach in the business world (see figure 7.2). It reflects a mentality of making a series of small improvements, evaluating the results each time, and making changes to improve the implementation. With health decisions, it means making a low-risk plan, putting it into action, and evaluating what worked and what didn't. Then tweak your approach before repeating the cycle. This method is great for situations where you're trying something new but want to proceed cautiously and adjust as you go.

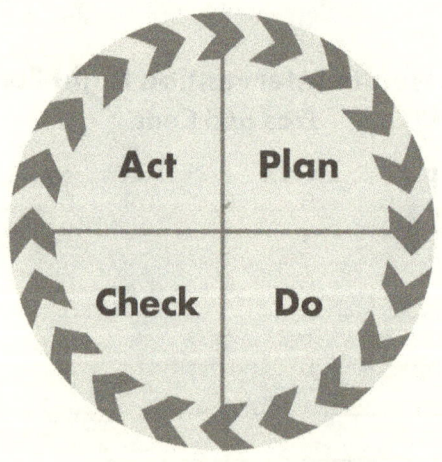

Figure 7.2: Plan-Do-Check-Act Cycle

3. **Force Field Analysis:** This is the more thoughtful cousin of the Pros and Cons List. Not only do you list the driving forces (reasons for) and restraining forces (reasons against), but you also assign weights to each factor (see the format in figure 7.3). This tool is perfect when you need to dig a little deeper and want to make sure

your decision aligns with your personal goals, values, and priorities. It's like getting a second opinion—from yourself!

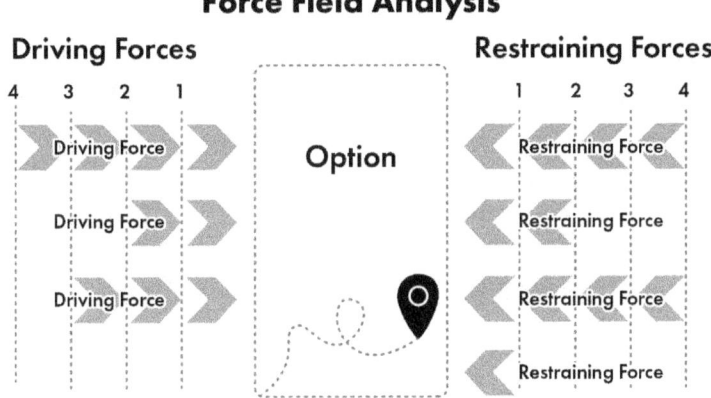

Figure 7.3: Force Field Analysis

4. **BRAIN Method:** If you're someone who likes to balance logic with gut feelings, the BRAIN Method is for you. This tool helps you list the **B**enefits, **R**isks, and **A**lternatives of a decision, then checks in with your **I**ntuition and assesses whether you **N**eed more time before deciding (see figure 7.4). It's ideal for those moments when you want to make sure your choice feels right in both your head and your heart. Take a few minutes before making a health decision and get your brain to go through the BRAIN Method to make sure you feel confident about your decision.

BRAIN Method

Benefits

Risks

Alternatives

Intuition

Need Time

Figure 7.4: The BRAIN Method

5. **Decision Matrix:** When you have multiple options and don't know how to choose, the Decision Matrix is a thorough way to go through the options. You list your options, identify the most important factors, and assign weights to each one. After some quick calculations, you'll see which option comes out on top (see figure 7.5). This method is perfect for complex decisions where you need to consider multiple factors and want to ensure you're making the most logical choice.

Decision Matrix

Important considerations					
Ranked on a scale of importance, with most importance associated with the highest number					
On a scale from 1 (least favorable) to 10 (most favorable), how well do the following solutions score based on the considerations above?					Total
Solution 1					
Solution 2					
Solution 3					
Solution 4					

Figure 7.5: Decision Matrix

Each tool provides a different perspective, helping us to evaluate options comprehensively. The Pros and Cons List clarifies the strengths and weaknesses of each choice, the PDCA Cycle supports gradual change, the Force Field Analysis offers a strategic overview, the BRAIN Method integrates intuitive and rational considerations, and the Decision Matrix provides a quantitative comparison.

Applying the Tools in Real Life

To illustrate how decision-making tools can improve the chance of successful health decisions, imagine Sarah, a thirty-five-year-old professional who has been struggling with weight management. She wants to lose weight but is overwhelmed by the options available. She is considering four options: (1) GLP-1 (glucagon-like peptide-1) medications, (2) weight loss surgery, (3) intermittent fasting, and (4) a thoughtful eating and exercise program. She values cost, has a moderate level of commitment, is high-risk tolerant, and desires effectiveness with minimal effort. She also prioritizes time, effort, and safety.

In the following section, I outline how each tool could guide Sarah toward a confident decision, helping her choose the weight loss method that best aligns with her needs and preferences. The tools are presented in the same order as before, starting with the simplest and progressing to the most complex.

Pros and Cons List

If Sarah doesn't feel the need to do a deeper analysis, she can simply create a Pros and Cons List for each option. She lists the advantages and disadvantages of GLP-1s, weight loss surgery, intermittent fasting, and the thoughtful eating and exercise program. By comparing these lists, she can see which method offers the best balance of benefits with manageable drawbacks. When looking at the lists, Sarah might find that each option offers unique advantages but also comes with potential drawbacks. GLP-1s and weight loss surgery promise significant weight loss, but Sarah is concerned about the potential side effects and the long-term commitment required for these interventions. Intermittent fasting appeals to her for its simplicity and effectiveness, but she worries about maintaining the routine with her unpredictable schedule.

In contrast, the thoughtful eating and exercise program emerges as the most balanced option for Sarah. While it requires effort and dedication, it doesn't carry the same risks as surgery or medication, and it's adaptable to her lifestyle. The program also allows her to make gradual, sustainable changes that align with her health goals without feeling overly restrictive.

By comparing these pros and cons (see figure 7.6), Sarah concludes that this approach offers the best combination of benefits with manageable challenges, making it the most suitable choice for her long-term health journey.

Is This Health Intervention Right For Me?
Pros and Cons List of GLP-1s for Weight Loss

Pros ↓	Cons ↓
Effective	Few long-term safety studies
Medical support	No end date for going off medications
Easy	Expensive, not covered by insurance
Appetite control	Potential side effects
	Weight gain after stopping medication
	I don't like to take shots

Figure 7.6: Example of a Pros and Cons List for Taking GLP-1s

Plan-Do-Check-Act (PDCA) Cycle

If Sarah were eager to get started or wanted to make sure that an option she had chosen is working out, she could start with small, manageable steps. She could set a goal to try intermittent fasting or a healthier diet for a month and incorporate additional minor lifestyle interventions into her routine, such as gradually reducing portion sizes and increasing her activity level. Each week she would review her *plan*, then *do* the plan (put it into action), *check* the results, and *act* to improve it—then implement the new plan and continue the cycle. This approach helps her ease into the process and build momentum without overwhelming herself.

Force Field Analysis

To identify which of the four options Sarah is considering has the most balanced benefits and challenges—and to help her narrow down which options are worth exploring further—she could do a Force Field Analysis for each option. She would list the driving forces (benefits of each method) and restraining forces (challenges or obstacles) for each option. For example, in Sarah's view, GLP-1s have the driving force of medical support and effectiveness but the restraining force of high cost (see figure 7.7). Weight loss surgery offers significant results but comes with high risk and recovery time.

In this case, the analysis revealed that the thoughtful eating and exercise program had strong driving forces, such as sustainability and adaptability, while its restraining forces, like effort and time commitment, were more manageable compared to the higher risks and costs of the other options.

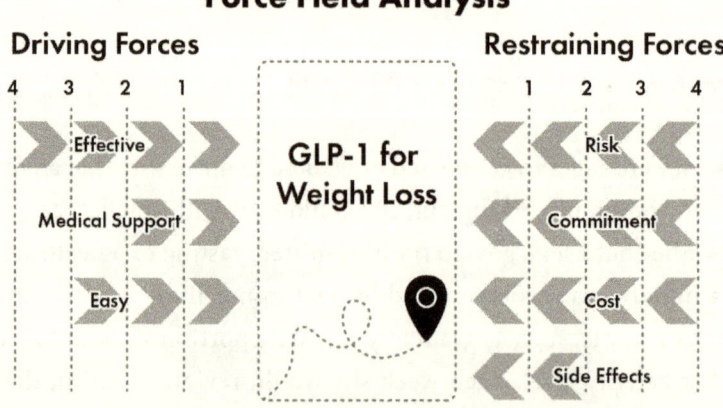

Figure 7.7: Example of Force Field Analysis

BRAIN Method

Alternatively, Sarah could analyze the benefits, risks, alternatives, intuition, and needed time (B-R-A-I-N) components for each of the options, which would allow her to take a holistic view of her options. By comparing the benefits of a controlled diet, such as health improvements and lower cost, against the risks of weight loss surgery, like surgical complications, she gains clarity on the potential outcomes of each choice.

Sarah's intuition tells her that a low-effort option like intermittent fasting might fit her lifestyle better, but through the BRAIN Method, she can balance these gut feelings with more concrete factors (see figure 7.8 for her BRAIN Method of using GLP-1s). For example, while intermittent fasting feels appealing, she might realize that the need time for adapting to this routine could conflict with her long-term goals. Ultimately, this method helps her make a well-rounded decision that accounts for both her practical needs and her personal instincts.

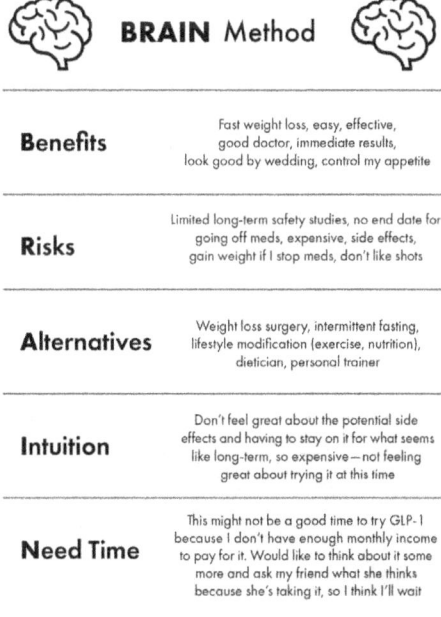

Figure 7.8: Example of a BRAIN Method

Decision Matrix

To help ensure that Sarah's analysis is objective and not swayed by biases or others' opinions, she could use a Decision Matrix to compare her options based on several criteria such as cost, effectiveness, effort required, and risk. This is the most complex of the tools listed because it considers factors that matter most to the person doing the analysis. In this matrix, each criterion is scored on a scale of 1 to 10, with 1 being the least favorable and 10 being the most favorable. Then, weights can be assigned to each criterion based on how important it is to Sarah. For example, Sarah may think cost matters more than effort, so she would assign a higher weight to cost.

Here are the four criteria chosen and how she defined them:

- **Cost**: This includes both the initial outlay of money (e.g., the cost of surgery) plus any additional expenses she would incur afterward (such as the cost of different foods if she changed her diet).
- **Effectiveness**: This measures how certain Sarah is that she will lose the weight she wants to lose.
- **Effort required**: This suggests how much effort on her part will be required to implement the option. For example, using drugs requires little effort on a daily basis compared to changing her exercise and eating habits.
- **Risk**: Sarah included both short-term and long-term risks in her assessment.

You can see the results of her decision-making in the following tables and figures. See table 7.1 for a description of the criteria Sarah used and the importance (or rank) that she assigned to each criterion. Table 7.2 summarizes the scores she assigned to each option based on a scale of 1 to 10, and table 7.3 shows the final outcome, where Sarah has multiplied the scores for each option by the weights for each criterion and come up with a final score.

Criteria	Cost	Effectiveness	Effort Required	Risk
Weights	2	4	1	3

Table 7.1: Criteria and Their Weights (Importance)

The criteria are considerations that matter most to Sarah. The weight is how much Sarah cares about each criterion, numbered in priority order (like a ranking of importance). She cares least about effort, so that is ranked #1, is slightly concerned about cost (#2), very concerned about risk (#3), and cares most about effectiveness (#4).

Option	Cost	Effectiveness	Effort Required	Risk	Score (before weighting)
Weight loss surgery	2	9	5	3	19
GLP-1s	4	8	8	7	27
Intermittent fasting	9	5	4	7	25
Thoughtful eating and exercise	7	8	5	8	28

Table 7.2: Initial Scoring (Without Weights)

Sarah scores each intervention in the four categories on a scale of 1 to 10, with 1 being the least favorable and 10 being the most favorable (meaning higher scores are better).

By the initial scoring, the thoughtful eating and exercise and taking GLP-1s are rated very similarly (27 vs. 28 respectively). Table 7.3 shows how the decision becomes clearer once the scores are weighted based on Sarah's priorities.

Option	Cost wt = 2	Effectiveness wt = 4	Effort Required wt = 1	Risk wt = 3	Total Score
Weight loss surgery	2 x 2 = 4	9 x 4 = 36	5 x 1 = 5	3 x 3 = 9	54
GLP-1s	4 x 2 = 8	8 x 4 = 32	8 x 1 = 8	7 x 3 = 21	69
Intermittent fasting	9 x 2 = 18	5 x 4 = 20	4 x 1 = 4	7 x 3 = 21	63
Thoughtful eating and exercise	7 x 2 = 14	8 x 4 = 32	5 x 1 = 5	8 x 3 = 24	75

Table 7.3: Weighted Scores
Sarah multiplies the weight number and the initial scores for each intervention. She then adds them up to come up with a total score.

You may disagree with Sarah's ratings, and that's okay. These tables reflect her decisions, and that's the point. She is documenting her decisions about these options.

Conclusion: Using the Decision Matrix makes Sarah's choice clear. Whereas GLP-1s and thoughtful eating and exercise were closely ranked without the weighting, now there is a clear separation *based on what is most important to her.* Thoughtful eating and exercise scores the highest overall at 75 due to its balance across all criteria, particularly in effectiveness and safety. Taking GLP-1s is much further behind. While her eating and exercise plan requires more effort than some other options, the manageable cost and strong performance in other areas make it the top choice for Sarah.

By utilizing tools like the Decision Matrix, Sarah—and anyone facing complex health decisions—can objectively weigh their options and make choices that align with their values and priorities. These tools not only provide clarity but also help ensure that decisions are well thought out and grounded in what matters most. As you move forward, it's essential to choose the decision-making method that best suits your unique situation, whether it's a straightforward comparison or a more detailed analysis. In the next section, we explore various decision-making methods to help you confidently navigate your health journey.

> ### Choosing a Decision-Making Method
>
> Here is my summary of when each tool is appropriate:
>
> - **Analytical decisions:** If your decision requires detailed analysis and you have time to weigh various factors, tools like Force Field Analysis and the Decision Matrix are ideal.
> - **Intuitive decisions:** When intuition plays a significant role and you need to balance it with logic, the BRAIN Method is your go-to tool.
> - **Feeling stuck:** If you're struggling to move forward and need to break the decision into smaller steps, the PDCA Cycle can help you make incremental progress.
> - **Quick decisions:** For fast decision-making without extensive deliberation, the Pros and Cons List provides a quick overview of potential outcomes.
>
> By choosing the right tool for your specific situation, you can ensure that your health decisions are thoughtful, well considered, and aligned with your goals and preferences. It also allows you to save time, money, and effort. In Sarah's case, by investing a few minutes to think through her options objectively, she could avoid making hasty decisions (as her personality tends to do) and can choose the most suitable path for her weight loss journey.

Leveraging Your Strengths

Understanding and leveraging your unique personality traits is key to making well-informed and effective health decisions. For example, a naturally analytical person might excel at researching treatment options, while a more empathetic, behavior-oriented individual might benefit from prioritizing supportive healthcare providers. Where you are strong in your decision-making, nurture those strengths and excel. Where you aren't, seek support or collaborate with others who complement your personality. The danger lies in thinking we can do it all—we all have strengths and weaknesses, and acknowledging this is a form of health humility.

As you navigate your health journey, remember that while your preferred approach to decision-making may remain consistent, different situations might call for different tools. Decision-making tools, such as the ones discussed earlier, can help you balance your natural tendencies with rational and efficient strategies. By integrating these tools into your process, you can break free from habitual patterns and make decisions that better align with your health goals.

Finally, it all comes back to embracing a mix of curiosity and humility. Staying open to new information and acknowledging the limits of your knowledge enhances your decision-making power. A higher health potential can be achieved at the intersection of leveraging the strengths of your personality, using smart decision-making tools, and always being curious and open to new ways of addressing health. Let's blow the cap off your healing capacity, shall we? If you believe it can happen, it will. Just keep reading.

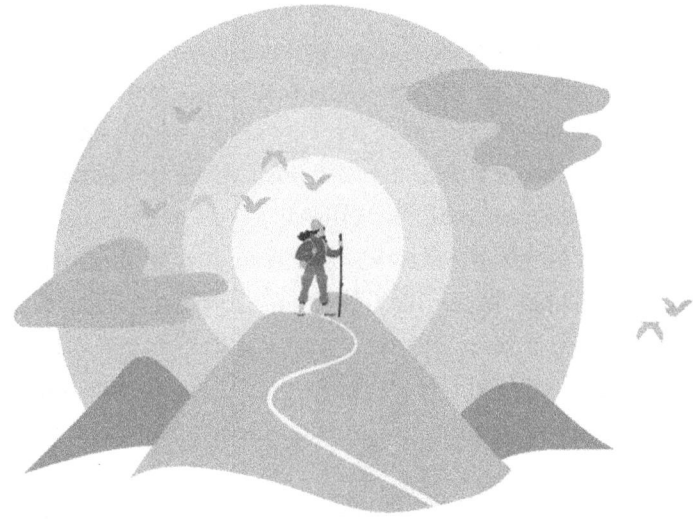

CHAPTER 8

Developing Confidence Through Belief and Attitude

If we're going to maximize our healing potential, we have to recognize the immense power of attitude and belief.

Every time we think about our health—whether it's deciding what to eat at a particular meal or choosing a path during a serious health crisis—our attitude plays a crucial role. Unlike personality traits, which are more fixed, our attitudes are something we can consciously shape. The way we choose to view our health challenges, not just deal with them, directly impacts our actions and, ultimately, our health outcomes.

Two people who face the same diagnosis can have completely different experiences based on their attitudes. One might approach the situation with fear and doubt, feeling overwhelmed by the obstacles ahead. The other, however, might choose to believe in their ability to heal, seeing the journey as an opportunity for growth and transformation. This belief not only boosts their confidence but also fuels their recovery. The difference? It's all in the attitude. As you navigate your health journey, the attitudes you adopt can either propel you forward or hold you back. By consciously choosing to cultivate a positive, empowering mindset, you unlock the potential to heal and thrive.

In fact, research supports this idea. A study published in the *Journal of Health Psychology* found that individuals with a positive attitude toward their health were more likely to engage in health-promoting behaviors, recover faster, and experience better overall health outcomes compared to those with a negative outlook.[1] Our mood and attitude are powerful in their capacity to impact our health.

Attitudes are complicated. They don't operate in isolation; they are shaped by many factors discussed in the preceding chapters, such as culture and circumstance. But in contrast to the personality traits discussed in the previous chapters, you *can* make conscious decisions about the attitudes you're going to adopt as you navigate health issues. We must believe and have the attitude that we can influence our healing capacity. Otherwise, we will miss out on potential healing.

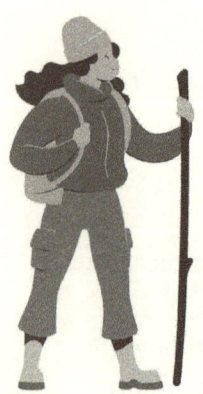

Our attitude and beliefs are like the weather shaping the landscape of our health.

The power of belief and attitude on health and healing cannot be overstated. Just as a positive mindset can boost your ability to recover, negative beliefs and expectations can have the opposite effect, potentially leading to illness. This phenomenon, known as the **nocebo effect**, shows that when we believe we won't recover or are destined to get a disease, those thoughts can manifest physically.[2]

Chronic stress, anxiety, and pessimism can weaken the immune system, increase inflammation, and disrupt the body's natural healing processes, making us more vulnerable to illness. Research has shown that people with a negative outlook on their health are more likely to experience adverse health outcomes, even when no underlying physical cause exists. This is why cultivating a positive belief in your ability to heal is so crucial—it's not just about optimism; it's about actively supporting your body's natural ability to stay healthy and recover.

Believing in yourself—often referred to as self-confidence—can be broken down into three key components: self-esteem, self-efficacy, and self-agency.

- Self-esteem reflects your overall sense of worth and how you value yourself.
- Self-efficacy is your belief in your ability to accomplish specific tasks and overcome challenges.
- Self-agency is the belief that you have control over your actions and the outcomes in your life.

Notice the key words in all three: *worth, value, belief, ability, control.* These words are powerful words that represent qualities everyone desires, and each one contributes something strong within us that allow us to navigate life with confidence and purpose. Together, these attitudes shape how you approach challenges, set goals, and persist in the face of obstacles. When you cultivate all three—self-esteem, self-efficacy, and self-agency—you're not just fostering a positive attitude; you're equipping yourself with the mindset needed to navigate health challenges and achieve success in various aspects of life.

All three—self-esteem, self-efficacy, and self-agency—offer us the opportunity to take ownership of our health and healing with confidence and renewed determination.[3] The stronger our belief in our ability to heal, the greater our chances of success. When we believe in ourselves, we build the confidence to take charge of our health. If we see ourselves as active participants in our health journey, rather than victims of circumstance, we're more likely to fulfill that belief and achieve better health outcomes. You can start to see how much power you have if you set your thinking to what you can do, and not what you can't. Let's explore these themes in more depth.

Self-Esteem: Believing in Yourself

Words and feelings provide valuable clues about where we stand on the spectrum of self-esteem. On one side, we have the realm of low self-esteem, where emotions like self-doubt, insecurity, and inadequacy tend to cast their shadows. These feelings, while challenging, can be crucial indicators, urging us to pay closer attention to the way we perceive ourselves and our health decisions. (See table 8.1.)

On the opposing side lies the territory of high self-esteem, illuminated by emotions like confidence, self-assuredness, and self-worth. These feelings not only uplift our spirits but also signify a strong foundation from which we can make positive health choices with conviction. By deciphering the subtle language of these emotions, we can better understand the role self-esteem plays in our Health Hero's journey and work toward fostering a mindset that propels us toward our wellness goals.

Examine the following words and discern where you resonate. Are you mostly within the realm of low or high self-esteem?

Low Self-Esteem	High Self-Esteem
Unhappy	Confident
Anxious	Neutral
Inferior	Capable
Impatient	Able
Resentful	Focused
Negative	Positive
Disinterested	Committed

Table 8.1: Low vs. High Self-Esteem

When our self-esteem is on the lower side, it can often feel like our well-being is under siege. In such moments, we might find ourselves inclined to give up quickly or lacking the necessary commitment to see our choices through.

For example, remember Terri from chapter 6? She'd decided that she needed to lose weight. If Terri decides to join a gym but carries low self-esteem when it comes to physical activity, she's more likely to struggle with regular attendance, fueled by her uncertainty.

On the other hand, if she had excessively high self-esteem when it comes to health decisions, that could manifest as overconfidence or a belief that she is invulnerable to health risks. People with overconfidence may disregard caution, fail to seek necessary medical advice, or engage in risky behaviors because they perceive themselves as infallible. To improve your self-esteem, here are some tips:

- **If you have low self-esteem:** To combat feelings of inadequacy, use positive self-talk where you challenge negative thoughts and replace them with positive, empowering self-talk. Be your own biggest supporter. Also, practice setting and achieving small, manageable goals; that will improve your confidence that you can accomplish goals. For example, if Terri decides to try a serene yoga class during her gym visit, she might be pleasantly surprised, with thoughts like, "I performed well in this yoga class, and I genuinely enjoyed it. I'll definitely give it another try."

- **If you suspect you may be overconfident:** Be curious! Even if you think you're right about something, embrace humility and seek out information or opinions from other sources and opinions. Even if turns out your initial idea was correct, you'll have more confidence by making informed and responsible choices.

Self-Efficacy: Belief in Your Ability

How confident are you in your ability to manage your health like a boss? Self-efficacy is all about our perceived competence in handling demanding situations, tackling difficult tasks, and, ultimately, reaching our objectives.

When our self-efficacy is soaring, we approach challenges with determination and persistence. We feel like we're in control of our health. It's like having an internal cheerleader urging us on. But when self-efficacy is lacking, we may hesitate to even start, or give up prematurely. You can see how in the case of Terri, the woman who wants to lose weight: If she believes she can successfully manage her weight, she's more likely to stay committed to her health journey. However, if she doubts her ability to make meaningful changes, it becomes an uphill battle. Table 8.2 shows a list of emotions she may feel depending on whether she has low or high self-efficacy.

Low Self-efficacy	High Self-Efficacy
Afraid of the risk	Confident in myself
Afraid of the uncertainty	Can evaluate the situation well
Concerned about failing	Willing to take risks
Pretending to be confident	Feel I can accomplish what I need to do

Table 8.2: Self-Efficacy

Self-efficacy isn't set in stone; it can be nurtured and developed over time. Setting achievable milestones, seeking guidance, and learning from past successes can significantly boost self-efficacy. For Terri, this might mean starting with small dietary adjustments, celebrating each victory, and gradually progressing to more ambitious health goals.

Let's say Terri generally feels uneasy about the idea of exercise, and her self-esteem in that area is quite low. Moreover, she doubts whether she could ever become someone who engages in regular physical activity because she doesn't possess the intrinsic motivation that she believes others have. Terri perceives herself as lacking proficiency in physical activity (related to self-esteem) and doubts her ability to become a physically active person (related to self-efficacy). In a scenario where Terri had high self-esteem, she might be more open to giving exercise a try, which could, in turn, boost her self-efficacy—these two factors can mutually influence each other. Alternatively, if Terri has low self-esteem but high self-efficacy, she might still go to the gym, albeit feeling uncomfortable, despite performing well in her fitness class.

Evaluating Your Own Self-Efficacy

What is your self-efficacy, Health Hero? To find out, complete the following sentences by inserting your health concern or the action you need to take to address it. Then, evaluate each statement on a scale of 1 (strongly disagree) to 5 (strongly agree), and calculate your total score afterward.

1. **I will be able to _____.**

(Example: I will be able to heal from cancer.)

2. **I am confident that I can perform _____ effectively to overcome my health challenge.**

(Example: I am confident that I can go through treatments to overcome cancer.)

3. **Compared to other people, I can overcome this health challenge very well.**

(Example: Compared to other people, I can face cancer very well.)

_____.

4. **Even with my health challenge and when times are tough, I will still perform well.**

(Example: Even with cancer and when times are tough, I will still do well.)

Add the scores from all four responses. Although results vary depending on the context of what you are assessing, if you score in a range between 16 and 20, this indicates a strong confidence in your abilities. You generally believe you can effectively overcome challenges and obstacles.

If your score is between 11 and 15, you have a moderate self-efficacy. You have some confidence in your abilities but may have some doubts or reservations about your capacity to achieve tasks or goals.

A score between 1 and 10 indicates low self-efficacy. You lack confidence in your abilities to accomplish tasks or goals related to your health concern. You may have significant barriers and doubt in your capacity to overcome these barriers.

After you've rated each statement on a scale of 1 to 5, you can then compare your total score to these descriptions. If your score falls within the range of 1 to 10, you might identify with some of the sentiments related to low self-efficacy.

On the other hand, if your score falls within the range of 16 to 20, you'll likely resonate with many of the feelings associated with high self-efficacy. This comparison can provide valuable insights into your self-perceived ability to take control of your health decisions. Remember, these descriptions are just a tool to help you gauge your self-efficacy, and your results can serve as a starting point for personal growth and development.

In the journey of becoming a Health Hero, understanding your self-efficacy is a crucial step. Your belief in your ability to make effective health decisions is not only an integral part of your story but also a powerful tool in shaping your narrative. Whether you've identified with low or high self-efficacy, remember that your self-perceived control over your health can be strengthened and refined. Recognize that it's okay to seek guidance, gather knowledge, and build your confidence as you embark on this path.

Here are several key strategies to strengthen your self-efficacy:

- **Be positive.** Try using positive self-talk and giving yourself grace to not be perfect.
- **Gather knowledge.** The more you know about your health and the options you're considering, the better you will be able to make good health decisions.
- **Visualize success.** Mentally rehearse success. Imagine yourself making healthy choices and experiencing positive outcomes.
- **Track your progress.** Keep a journal or record of your health decisions and their results or try using health tracking apps. I discuss tracking in later chapters and provide tracking sheets. Seeing your progress will boost your self-efficacy.
- **Seek support.** Engage with a mentor, health coach, or support group to guide and encourage you on your journey. It's important to have allies!
- **Learn from setbacks.** Don't be discouraged by failures or setbacks. Instead, view them as opportunities to learn and grow. Easier said than done, but it's true.
- **Celebrate achievements.** Recognize and celebrate your successes, no matter how small they may seem. This reinforces your belief in your ability to make health-conscious decisions.
- **Pray.** Prayer can boost self-efficacy by providing a sense of support, inner strength, and resilience. You feel more confident

in your abilities when you believe a higher power is helping you. Prayer and belief in God offer a source of guidance, clarity, and empowerment. Here is an example of a Christian prayer to bring immediate confidence. Feel free to make one of your own.

Dear Lord, You command us to go in confidence and face whatever is ahead of us because You are by our side. I pray that You stay by my side as I improve my health. Help me to live without fear or hesitation today with the knowledge that You are with me. Be my cheerleader who encourages me. Give me strength and power to heal and recover. In Jesus's name, Amen.

- **Take action.** The more you practice making health decisions, the more confident you'll become. Action builds self-efficacy.
- **Be patient.** Building self-efficacy is a process that takes time. Be patient with yourself as you develop this empowering attribute.

You, Health Hero, are capable of achieving mighty health goals. By implementing these strategies, you can gain the confidence you need to get healthy and achieve more than you ever imagined.

Self-Agency: Believing You Have Control over Your Circumstances

To what extent do you believe you have the power to steer your health journey in the right direction? In other words, do you perceive life and external factors as obstacles or as allies in your pursuit of health? Self-agency is the belief that we can make progress in spite of our environment and circumstances, can overcome health adversaries, and that we have control over our health destiny. When we possess low self-agency, it may seem as if unfavorable events, like declining health or limited access to resources, are beyond our control. Conversely, individuals with high self-agency maintain a confident attitude, believing they can and will find a way to take the necessary actions to improve their health and seek the resources they need for recovery.

Let's look at Terri again and compare what she'd be like with low self-agency and high self-agency (see table 8.3).

Terri with Low Self-Agency	Terri with High Self-Agency
I can't exercise, because the gyms don't accommodate people who aren't in shape.	I will find ways to get in shape at the gym that don't embarrass me.
The gym doesn't have classes for people like me.	I will try different classes and find a class that suits me.
I don't know what exercises to do and how much to do them.	I will hire a personal trainer to help me figure out what I need to do.
I will slip and stop going to the gym over the holidays.	I will be persistent in going to the gym by making weekly goals.
Exercise hurts too much.	I will get stronger once I get used to moving again.

Table 8.3: Example of Low vs. High Self-Agency

I talk about medical disclaimers in chapter 3, but what I didn't mention was how they can take away your self-agency. Medical disclaimers, while important for legal and safety reasons, can sometimes have the unintended effect of undermining our sense of ability to make our own decisions. By constantly reminding us to seek professional advice for every health decision, they can make us feel powerless or overly dependent on external authorities. This can rob us of the confidence to trust our instincts and make informed choices about our own health. In essence, while these disclaimers aim to protect, they can also inadvertently strip away our personal empowerment, leaving us feeling like passive participants in our health journey rather than active, capable decision-makers. Don't be afraid to make your own health decisions. Use common sense when seeking medical advice. You have more control over your health than anyone.

Improving Self-Agency

While the practices previously listed for enhancing self-esteem and self-efficacy also contribute to building self-agency, the single most important step you can take to build self-agency is to **take action**. Any positive action will do. Be consistent and track your progress over a set period of time. This process of doing, tracking, and seeing progress will strengthen your belief in your ability to influence your health and wellness, guaranteed. Each positive step you take builds a sense of control and empowerment.

Don't know where to begin? Here are some no-cost, straightforward goals to get you started that you can easily achieve, no matter what your circumstance are:

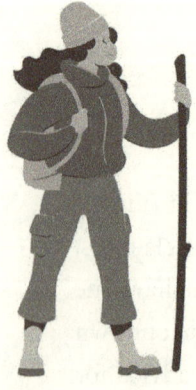

Disclaimers instill fear, but awareness makes our path clear.

- **Stay hydrated.** Aim to drink an adequate amount of water daily. Start by carrying a reusable water bottle and setting reminders to take sips throughout the day. This simple habit can boost energy and overall well-being and make you feel like you accomplished something big.

- **Take short walks.** Incorporate short walks into daily routines. Take a ten-minute walk during a break at work or after dinner. Walking is an excellent way to exercise without feeling overwhelmed.

- **Practice mindful eating.** Choose one meal a day and make the effort to savor each bite, eat without distractions, and pay attention to hunger and fullness cues. Listen to your body and tune into your emotions to see how they respond to the food.
- **Set a nurturing bedtime routine.** Establish a bedtime routine that promotes relaxation, such as reading or gentle stretching, and track improvements in your sleep.
- **Prepare meals.** Plan and prepare one healthy meal a week. Preparing a home-cooked meal allows for better control over ingredients and portion sizes. The key word is control—you control what you cook and eat. You get to make all of the decisions.

These achievable goals are small steps that can lead to more significant changes in your health. They will help you realize that you have more power over your health than you previously thought. Circumstances may overwhelm you, *but you still have control over your actions.*

Remember, even small actions can lead to significant changes over time. Don't wait for the perfect moment—start today.

Better Health Through a Positive Attitude

Because both we and our circumstances can get in the way of our attitude, we have to accept that all three attitudes I just discussed—self-esteem, self-efficacy, and self-agency—will fluctuate. What might appear as low self-esteem one evening could transform after a good night's rest. Rather than assuming that your current attitude is your permanent perspective, pause for a moment to reflect on how you typically approach different aspects of your life. Is this attitude a recent development, or does it align with your typical personality tendencies? Be fully

continued

> honest with yourself. If you are, you'll know when an attitude adjustment is needed, or when you just need some self-care.

Reinforce Your Spirituality

I would be remiss if I failed to talk about a critical factor that strongly impacts your health that you have control over, yet probably seldom think about. What is this? It's how much you choose to believe in the transformative influence of what is beyond human, a higher power, on the journey to healing.

There is no minimizing the impact of prayer and spirituality on health. Studies suggest that prayer and spirituality can reduce stress, improve mental well-being, enhance recovery from illness or surgery, and even increase our chances of living longer.[4] Even Carl Gustav Jung, a pioneer of modern psychology, emphasized the importance of spirituality on our well-being, saying, "Every crisis over the age of thirty is a spiritual crisis. Spiritual crises require spiritual cures."

This spiritual connection, this unwavering faith, is not just a matter of the soul; it's a profound force that ripples through the body and the mind, nurturing the healing process. It whispers solace in times of uncertainty, ignites hope in the face of adversity, and weaves a protective armor of emotional resilience.

Our belief in something greater than ourselves serves as a guiding light, offering both solace and strength as we navigate the turbulent waters of health challenges. It is a reminder that, in our quest for wellness, we are not alone; we are part of a greater, divine tapestry. This sacred connection, in the Health Hero's world, is a source of comfort, resilience, and a profound understanding of the interconnected nature of body, mind, and spirit, fostering not just healing but also an enduring sense of purpose.

You have this power, too, and it's important to recognize how spirituality can expand our human healing possibilities. Flexing spiritual muscles moves us from a place of spiritual potential to spiritual health, much like choosing to exercise or eat nutritiously. If you want to maximize your health, expand your spirituality.

Healing Mantras: The Juncture of Esteem, Efficacy, Agency, and Spirituality

The mind-body connection plays a powerful role in our healing journey, and setting positive health intentions can significantly influence our outcomes. Research has shown that the more we believe in our ability to heal, the better our chances of recovery. Studies in psychology and neuroscience suggest that positive affirmations and beliefs can reduce stress, improve mental health, and even enhance physical healing. By repeating healing mantras, you reinforce these positive beliefs, allowing them to ingrain in your thinking and guide your actions toward recovery.

Healing mantras are simple yet powerful phrases that you can repeat daily to set your intentions and align your mind with your healing goals. These affirmations remind you of your body's innate ability to recover and strengthen your resolve to overcome health challenges. For example, you might say, "I am resilient and will rise above this health challenge," or "I can determine my health destiny through faith and belief." Another powerful mantra could be, "My body is equipped to heal, so I believe it will heal." By integrating these mantras into your daily routine, you foster a mindset of hope and determination, which can positively impact your healing process.

The science behind this is compelling. Studies on the placebo effect, for instance, demonstrate that belief in a treatment's effectiveness can lead to real physiological improvements, even when the treatment is inactive.[5] Similarly, research on mindfulness and positive psychology shows that optimistic thinking can reduce inflammation, enhance immune function, and improve overall well-being.[6] By consistently focusing on positive, healing thoughts, you're not only shaping your mindset but also creating fertile ground for your body to heal.

Incorporating healing mantras into your health strategy is a simple yet effective way to reinforce your belief in your ability to recover. Repeat these phrases throughout your day—whether during meditation, before sleep, or whenever you need a boost of confidence. Over time, these affirmations can help shift your mindset from uncertainty to empowerment, strengthening your commitment to your healing journey.

Do You Believe You Can Heal?

Ultimately, the topics in this chapter come down to one critical question: **Do you believe you can heal?** If you haven't thought about it much, it's time.

We all have an inner critic to contend with, and sometimes it shows up when we have health concerns. We experience self-doubt, self-criticism, or self-berating, and it can sound like, "You shouldn't spend that much money on your health!" or "Trying that intervention is stupid—it's not going to work."

I've come to think of this voice as the part of us who wants to protect us. It's the part of us that cares deeply and wants us to do things the right way. But there is no right way by definition—the right way to manage our health is by doing our best. To do this, there is no exact approach or method. It is flexible and experimental. Your inner critic needs to be gently reassigned to stepping back and quieting down.

You, Health Hero, don't have time to entertain your inner critic. If your inner critic is speaking loudly to you, gently thank it, and then tell it to calm down and trust the Health Hero within you. You are more than capable of moving through this health issue without the inner critique interjecting doubt. As a matter of fact, your inner critic is taking up valuable time that could be using to research and strategize ways to heal.

There is nothing wrong with how you are approaching your health issue. You are more than enough to handle whatever comes your way. Trust me, trust you, and trust your body.

You possess tremendous, yet often underutilized, power to shape yourself and your health. It all rests on your attitude. Shift your attitude to propel you forward, not hold you back, and you'll break free from the grip of helplessness.

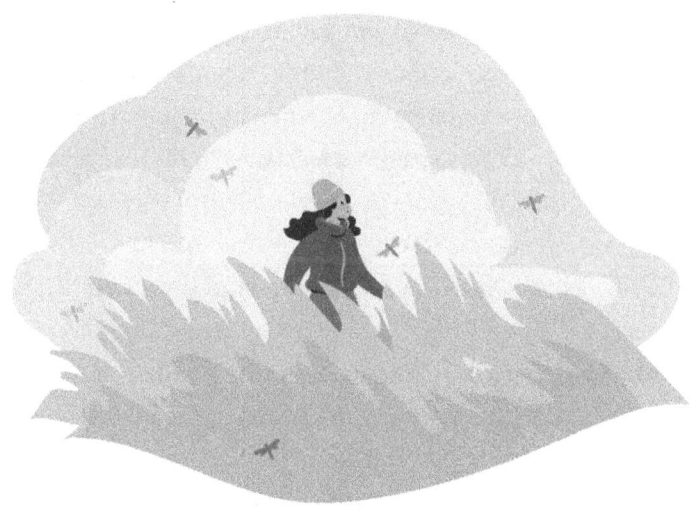

CHAPTER 9

Naming the Unnamed: Being Able to Articulate Your Emotions

My client Julia called me in a panic—her doctor told her that she had breast cancer. As she shared her story, she told me she was worried and felt fragile, overwhelmed, panicky, lost, lonely, and even angry. Can you imagine how unnerving it would feel to get such news? You actually may have been, or are, in her shoes this very minute. If you are, I want to first stop and give you permission to feel. Health concerns release all kinds of feelings, from sorrow to feeling betrayed. Your feelings matter. I want to encourage you to feel deeply about your health situation.

Because of our emotions, no health journey will ever be a perfectly logical, straightforward series of choices, but rather an erratic display of behaviors. We feel courage one minute, and anxiety and worry the next. Because health is so personal and so vital to our future, most of us take it seriously. Maybe too seriously at times. On the other hand, we sometimes turn off our emotions completely and become apathetic. Often our emotions abate, leaving us without a catalyst to move in any direction to find better health. Whether you overreact or underreact, emotions are driving your next health action.

That is why it is important to understand the emotional whirlwind we experience around our health, so we can continue to stand strong and walk toward healing regardless of our feelings, or we can change how we feel to drive us toward faster healing. Addressing health without addressing emotions is like taking away Picasso's soul and expecting him to paint a masterpiece. It would not have been possible.

But more than that, I want you to name those feelings because it will help. Let me show you how and tell you why it might save your life.

Getting Grounded Through Emotional Storms

There are many advantages of being aware of your emotional state with the help of the emotion wheel.[1] Here are some of the most obvious ones.

Recognizing emotions can give you a jump start on taking care of potentially dangerous health issues. I've had many clients sense something wasn't quite right long before the medical tests found anything wrong. They described it as a feeling of guilt, unsettledness, or uneasiness. Your body uses emotions to communicate, so if you're listening, you can start to hear it give you a nudge to stop a behavior that's not healthy or add a health behavior that helps it heal. This can feel like intuition or a gut feeling—there's nothing to prove it, but you just *know*. When this happens, you can seek medical advice or keep tabs on the feeling to see if it changes after implementing some healthy lifestyle interventions, like drinking more water, getting more sleep, eating healthier foods, or exercising.

You can start to recognize emotional patterns and plan ahead. Perhaps you track your daily emotions for a week and notice that you're irritable every day at around 3:30. You can start to implement some strategies that might help, like taking a walk at that time, or eating a small, healthy snack. Or maybe you take a five-minute break and do some deep-breathing exercises or meditation. You can notice associations between your emotions and outside circumstances. Maybe your irritability comes from a bombardment of emails from a coworker. Or maybe it's the time of day you realize that you didn't get all you wanted to do done, so you begin to stress. Patterns are powerful—they can give you insight into what's not working well for your mental and physical health.

Knowing your emotions can be used as a tool for encouragement. Noticing when negative feelings have crept up in similar past circumstances can give you much-needed perspective. Perhaps you have had past situations when similar emotions appeared, yet to your relief you experienced health turnarounds in spite of those emotions. "I've noticed these feelings before—it was when I had my last health scare! I made it through that time, so I am confident I can make it through this situation, too."

For example, I've had many a night where I only got a couple of hours of sleep and the next day felt anxious and fearful. Knowing that I have this pattern tendency has helped me recognize that if I don't get a good night's sleep, I will likely get anxious or paranoid, and that the feelings are only temporary.

Being aware of how you manifest emotions can also help you from making irrational decisions. Many times, our emotions get in the way of our actions. I've had clients take handfuls of pain medications because they overreacted from a pain or sprain. If you want to do your best to make the most logical health decision, and you want to feel in control and capable of overcoming the health challenge, manage your emotions and don't make a big decision until you clear your head. A clear head leads to good decisions, and good decisions lead to faster healing. If you've ever been in a situation where you can't seem to manage your emotions, don't do anything yet until you ask someone for their perspective. Ask someone you trust to verify if what you're going to do sounds appropriate. If my client would have asked me if they should take all those medications, I would have tried to calm them down and talk them out of it. Sometimes it takes an outside perspective to keep us from mismanaging our health.

Emotions can be your body's way of telling you to rest. Have you ever felt continually overwhelmed just before coming down with a cold or flu? Or have you felt like your injury won't heal? It might be your body's way of saying, "Slow down; you need to rest. I'm trying to recover or fight off this infection."

Understanding that emotional fluctuations are natural can reduce stress. Emotional fluctuations are a natural part of life. Many women, for instance, can anticipate changes in their mood associated with their menstrual cycle. Similarly, seasonal changes affect the mood of many individuals. Moods can often be cyclical and somewhat predictable. By tracking our moods and emotions, we can gain relief from understanding that what we're feeling is not only real but also expected and predictable. Recognizing these patterns reassures us that we're not "going crazy"—our emotions are simply following their normal course. By identifying these patterns, we can implement strategies to manage our emotions proactively before they become overwhelming.

Recognizing our feelings also helps us show ourselves empathy. When we're feeling down and discouraged, it might be time to give ourselves grace and space to nurture our spirits with activities we enjoy and that bring us joy.

One of the most important reasons to pay attention to your emotions is to recognize when they might be leading you astray. It's instinctive to want to react to your emotions: if you're angry, you might feel like throwing something; if you're upset, you may want to say something you don't mean. When you're sick, reactions can vary. Since we all react differently, it's beneficial to start recognizing our default reactions by using tools like the emotion wheel. Understand how your feelings manifest themselves with actions. Appeal to your rational self, rather than your emotions, and you will be better able to make better health decisions and recover more quickly.

What I Am Feeling: The Emotion Wheel

When you hear the word *cancer* come from your doctor's mouth, first get diagnosed with something serious, or even when you suspect that you might be up against a serious health concern, strong or new feelings begin to emerge. Will I live? Am I going to have to go through chemo? Will I be able to participate in my favorite activities?

Sometimes these feelings can be intense, while at other times they show up as subtle shifts in mood, or a sense of feeling off. It is at this time that Health Heroes can be strategic and use their feelings to propel them forward to healing.

Feelings are sometimes hard to describe, so I use the emotion wheel (figure 9.1) to help my clients sort through their emotions. This clever tool breaks down feelings into three levels that allow them to dial-in their emotions so they can easily find and name their feelings.

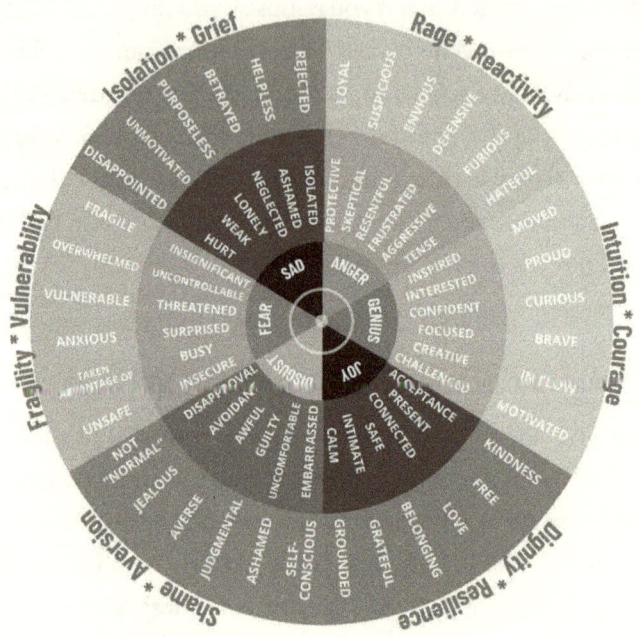

Figure 9.1: The Emotion Wheel

If you've never seen an emotion wheel, it looks similar to a color wheel that artists and painters use. It's made up of three layered, concentric circles representing different levels of emotions.

1. The inner layer represents **primary emotions,** which are general emotions such as happiness, sadness, anger, and fear.

2. The middle layer represents the **secondary emotions** that stem from the primary emotions. These emotions home in our feelings a little more precisely so that we can start to drill down past the primary emotion to a more precise word.

3. The third, outer layer represents the **tertiary emotions,** which are an even further breakdown of the secondary emotions. These

words can continue to help you tease out the crux of the feeling if the secondary emotions aren't hitting the mark.

For example, let's say Julia felt fear after hearing about her cancer diagnosis. That primary emotion of fear at the core of the wheel can manifest itself in a variety of ways. She may, for example, feel threatened, worried, insecure, and/or fragile. Feeling more than one secondary emotion with each primary emotion is completely natural. These feelings may ultimately make her feel anxious, terrified, unsafe, or vulnerable, using the words in the outermost layer.

Now, here's how being able to put labels on your feelings is helpful: once you have a word describing more precisely how you feel, ask yourself what it is that's causing you to feel that way and what you could do to feel differently. For example, if you feel fear, and more precisely, insecure, why is that? Is it because you don't feel like you have the resources to overcome your health issue? Or is it because you don't feel sure you can psychologically make it through this scary situation? Finding resources to help with either would be different, so it's helpful to know the difference. For the fear of lack of resources, the solution would be connecting you to different resources that might help (information, funding, health assistance, etc.). For the fear of not being able to face the challenge of going through a health scare, the solution might be getting emotional support resources to help you cope with your strong feelings. Once you define the words, you can start to strategize how to overcome the root feeling behind them.

Mood Matters

Back again to Julia. What did I do next to help her figure out what to do with her breast cancer diagnosis? I bet it's not what you think I would do, which is to dive into the treatment and

continued

> healing intervention options. No, the first thing I did for Julia was to shift her mood, and now you know why. Mood matters.
>
> Like I said before, your mood impacts your health decisions. If you want to make good health decisions, shift your mood. The emotion wheel can help you find feelings that evoke the feeling you desire, such as positive, empowering, and motivational. What positive emotions do you want to embody as you navigate your health issue? How about trying these: motivated, brave, curious, inspired, or confident. Find the right words that inspire you.

Tips for a Positive Outlook During Health Challenges

To overcome overpowering emotions, I've created some mental practices to build up the emotional strength muscle. Practice them often so you can become emotionally prepared for any health issue that comes your way. Try them out to see which ones bring about a calmer mood and a better sense of control for you during times of emotional distress, in particular around health issues.

Research and gather evidence. Look for evidence of positive outcomes for your health condition. For example, Julia's cancer was detected early, and based on the latest evidence, her five-year survival rate was about 99 percent. Knowing this significantly improved her outlook.

Find inspirational stories. Seek out stories of people who have successfully navigated similar health issues. This could involve meeting someone to hear about their experience or reading an article or book. Knowing that others have overcome similar challenges can boost your positivity.

Engage with your spirituality. Whether through prayer or seeking a higher power, connecting with your spiritual side can be comforting. Julia and I, both Christians, prayed together and entrusted her healing to Jesus, which helped her feel less alone and more hopeful. This approach can be adapted to any spiritual belief, helping to shift your mood from fear to trust and hope.

Surround yourself with positive people. Seek out the positive individuals in your life who can lift your mood. Positive people are invaluable because they bring hope and encouragement. While life isn't always perfect, a dose of positivity can be very helpful. If you can't find anyone positive around you, reach out to me, and I'll encourage you or connect you with one of my coaches. In my experience, health coaches are naturally great encouragers.

Implementing these strategies can help improve your mental and emotional well-being during challenging health situations. Emotions aren't our enemy; they exist to protect us and help us navigate our circumstances. Approach the emotions you're feeling by embracing them with curiosity, and ultimately, love. Then gently nudge them to help you move in a better direction by focusing on positive emotions, not negative ones. Emotions are the windshield through which we view the world, and we want our windshield to have a clear view so that we can drive quickly down the road to recovery.

Putting Emotional Intelligence to Work

I've just given you some rich knowledge in managing your emotions through health challenges. Congratulations—you just learned about one of the two parts of the emotional intelligence equation. The first part of emotional intelligence is the ability to recognize, understand, and manage *your own* emotions. The other half is the ability to recognize and understand the emotions of *others*, so you can better manage your response to them and perhaps find insights into their reactions that will help you understand your situation more deeply.

Why does it help to be aware of others' emotions as it relates to managing your health? First, many times, other people's emotions rub off on us, affecting our feelings and decisions. I know that when I'm with someone who is worried about my health, then I become more worried about my health, more than I was before. Knowing this can happen allows you to offset by employing strategies like setting boundaries, establishing your desired mindset, practicing critical thinking, and focusing on guarding your feelings to maintain emotional balance. Learn when to walk away from people who negatively influence your thinking and toward people who enhance it.

With emotional intelligence, we can also view our healthcare providers' frustrations or annoyance objectively, understanding their emotions without letting it negatively impact our perception or decisions (or helps us know when to get a new provider). Or, if our doctor has empathy and is hopeful about our health outcome, we can lean in and take comfort in their care.

Embrace ALL Your Emotions

It's not only okay to take some time and "feel the yucky feelings," it's important to do that because, as I mentioned before, feelings are another way your body communicates to you. Your feelings are trying to relay a message. You won't likely be able to fix the issue in an instant, so instead, think in a way that prompts you to overcome and move forward.

Acknowledge your feelings by telling them that you hear them loud and clear. They've done their job to get you spurred to address the concern, so they can now start to subside, and you can then turn on new feelings that are more positive and encouraging—or at the very least not panic inducing. How do I know this? I've taken research from sports psychologists and athletic success. Studies show that within a group of athletes of equal ability, those who receive mental training (psychological awareness) outperform those who don't almost every time.[2] Emotions happen to the best of athletes, but those who learn to manage their emotions win. But like physical skills, emotional skills can only be developed through constant practice. You may not be able to control everything about your health concern, but you can control your emotions. One of the most important things you can do to manage your health is to manage what's above your shoulders—your thoughts and your head.

Keep in mind, too, that developing emotional intelligence not only helps you navigate your own emotional landscape but also equips you to better understand and respond to the emotional cues of those around you. Take confidence from knowing that you can handle anything or anyone that comes your way because you are emotionally prepared.

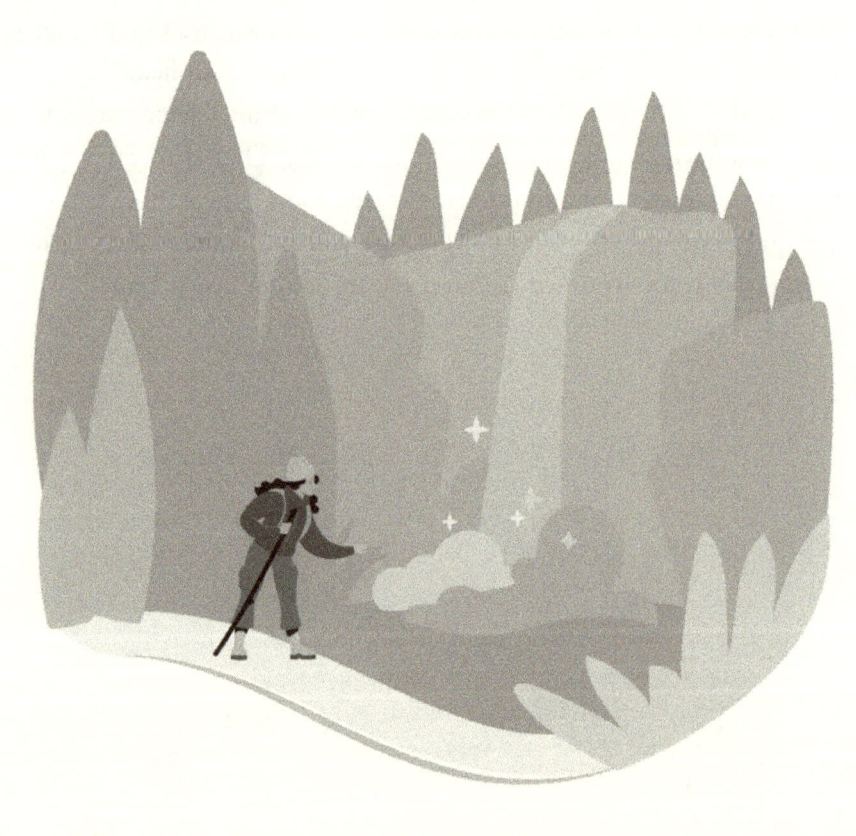

Part III

Making Healing Happen: Your Action Plan

Now that you've deepened your self-awareness and identified the internal and external forces affecting your health, it's time to turn that insight into action. In this section, we transform your newfound clarity into a personalized, actionable plan that guides you toward faster, sustainable healing. Part III empowers you to take control of your health journey with confidence, clarity, and purpose, equipping you with the tools and strategies necessary to meet any challenge.

Together, we map out a comprehensive approach to your health by

- developing a clear, detailed understanding of your current health status and how it should be the foundation of your decisions (chapter 10);
- defining a health approach that aligns with your personal goals and values (chapter 11);
- exploring the Core 4 lifestyle interventions that form the cornerstone of well-being (chapter 12);
- discovering additional lifestyle interventions that can enhance your healing journey (chapter 13);
- understanding the role of conventional medicine to prevent unmet expectations and maximize its strengths (chapter 14);

- discovering the benefits of complementary practices and a blended approach to healing (chapter 15); and
- crafting a tailored Healing Action Plan that will support you through any health situation, no matter how complex (chapter 16).

If you're ready to step into the role of your own Health Hero and embrace the path to faster healing, let's begin.

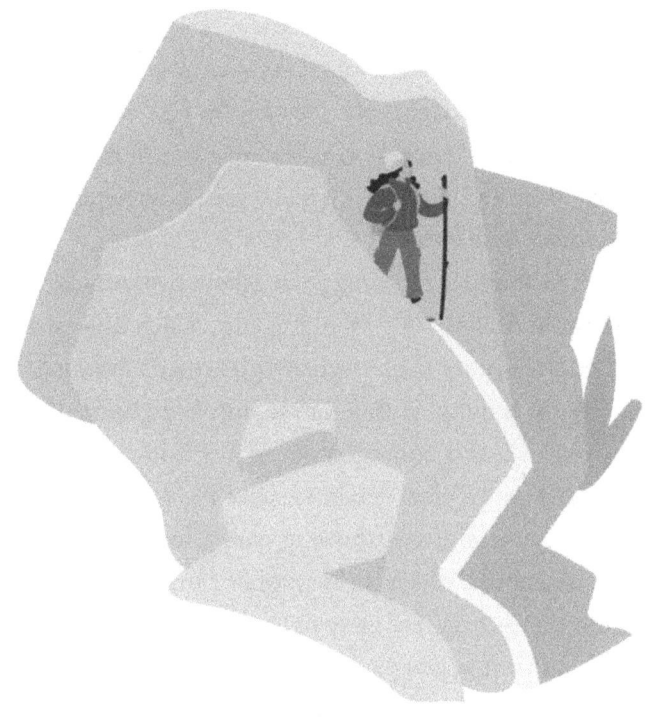

CHAPTER 10

How Is Your Health . . . Really?

Kristen, one of my clients, now enjoys an enviable physique and boundless energy—but that wasn't always the case. When she first came to me, she was struggling with excess weight and constant fatigue. Determined to get "in shape," she reached out for guidance. Early in our journey, I encouraged her to start with a comprehensive health assessment, a key step in the health awareness process. The results were a wake-up call—elevated blood pressure, blood sugar, and cholesterol levels. She was both surprised and disheartened by what she learned.

She soon realized that her weight gain was accompanied by other silent conditions lurking beneath the surface.

"What are these results about?" Kristen asked, visibly concerned. "Sure, I'm a bit overweight, but I generally take care of myself. I eat well. Maybe I could include more cardio exercise in my routine, but this shouldn't be." Her declining health had crept up on her over the past few years, taking her by surprise.

Together, we traced the turning point. About two years ago, she'd started a new job while dealing with marital issues, which unleashed a wave of uncontrolled stress, poor sleep, overeating, excessive drinking, and a sharp drop in physical activity. With a family history of heart disease, Kristen was already at risk, and under that stress, her body began to respond in ways she hadn't anticipated. When we have a genetic predisposition, our bodies often react to stress by showing symptoms in that vulnerable area. In my case, it's asthma, which flares up when I'm under stress. For Kristen, the mounting stress triggered early signs of heart disease.

What about you? When you're under stress, do you notice symptoms that hit your body's genetic weak spots?

Kristen's heart disease was difficult to detect from the outside. Symptoms like breathlessness and fatigue were quickly dismissed as simply being out of shape. This is where blood work became invaluable—it uncovered the hidden health issues beneath the surface. Her life circumstances, combined with these findings, made it clear that immediate action was necessary to reclaim her health.

Kristen's story is typical: many of us go through life unaware of what's happening to our health. We get accustomed to stress, poor eating habits, and inactivity, living in the moment without realizing the impact on our bodies.

For example, consider what happens when we eat fast food. A meal like a cheeseburger and fries causes our blood fat levels to spike within minutes and stay elevated for hours. I often saw this firsthand while working at a company that offered blood screenings. Patients who ate unhealthy meals the night before would have cloudy, dense plasma instead of the clear fluid expected in a healthy person. Their lab results consistently showed elevated cholesterol and triglycerides.

Our blood tells the real story. Just one fatty meal or one sugary treat strains the body, forcing it to clear out excess fat and sugar to prevent long-term cell damage. Repeated assaults, like meal after meal of fast food, eventually lead to severe conditions like heart disease, stroke, and diabetes. And once diseases like diabetes take hold, they can be costly and difficult to manage.

Without a full, honest assessment of our health—whether through physical symptoms or medical evaluations like blood work—we risk continuing harmful habits without realizing it. We often manage our health on autopilot, unaware that we could perpetuate patterns that undermine our well-being.

The good news is that our bodies are constantly communicating with us. Whether through dips in energy, aches, discomfort, or changes we may not immediately notice—like shifts in our blood markers—these are all signals urging us to pay attention. Blood work, for instance, provides an inside look at how our body is functioning, revealing imbalances or potential issues before they manifest as physical symptoms. By tuning in to both the subtle messages of our body and the insights gained through medical assessments, we can take meaningful action before our health concerns become chronic.

I encourage you to actively listen to your body's external and internal signals. In the following sections, I guide you through how to do just that, but first, let's take a moment to get honest about where your health stands today.

Let's Face It: Your Body Yesterday Was Not What It Is Today

When it comes to our health, we are constantly changing. We grow, mature, age, and endure health challenges. As we navigate life, we get injured and become slightly less resilient as we move through midlife.

Our health management evolves as we get busier. We change, so our health changes.

Many people rely on their past health to justify their current state: "I've always been healthy," "I'm athletic," "I'm in good shape," "I've never had health issues. . . ." We remember ourselves at our peak condition. But that was yesterday, not today. Our bodies change as our lives adapt to new demands and circumstances. Sometimes, our bodies temporarily adjust and return to their previous state, but more often, we settle into a new normal of health. We must accept our health where we are *now*, not where we *were*, and we need to pay attention to our health to appreciate the differences.

The key is recognizing our current health state and knowing when to intervene. By paying close attention, we can identify signs, symptoms, or subtle changes before they become problematic. Awareness is a powerful tool to prevent health issues from escalating to the point where minor adjustments and interventions are no longer sufficient. You will catch health issues early if you build awareness into your regular health routine.

There are two powerful ways to uncover your actual health status. The first is by identifying your specific pain points—both obvious and subtle. Sometimes your body screams, sometimes it talks, and sometimes it only whispers. If you listen closely, you'll be amazed at what it reveals. The second is through objective assessment, and I've created a tool to help with that. Let's begin by exploring your aches, pains, and discomforts. Please, promise to stay open and curious about what your body has to share as you explore your health status. Remember, knowledge is power, and you're about to gain some serious power by acquiring knowledge about your health.

Pain Points: Where Does It Hurt?

Typically, I encourage thinking of your body as a whole—where mind and body are interconnected—for a balanced approach to health.

However, when it comes to health awareness, I'm going to ask you to think differently. Instead of seeing the body as a whole, consider it in parts. Each part has built-in indicators, much like gauges on a car dashboard, providing valuable information. Let's take a look at the dashboard of your health by conducting a short scan of your body.

- Start by taking a minute to be quiet and relaxed. Breathe deeply and let your muscles loosen.
- Ask yourself how you feel—both physically and mentally.
- Then, ask your body to reveal any pain. Methodically move your awareness slowly from the top of your body down, and from the left of your body to the right, from inside out, and from front to back.
- As you move from body section to body section, note any discomfort or new sensation, such as tingling, tension, ringing in your ears, or warmth. Notice any sensations or areas of pain, discomfort, or imbalance. Notice all your senses: touch, smell, sight, hearing, and taste. Do things seem brighter to you lately? Have you lost your sense of taste or smell? Is your mouth dry? Do your shoulders feel tight? How do your feet feel?
- Now think about how you've moved through the world lately. Do you feel like you've lost balance, or do you get dizzy when you turn your head to the left? Think about pain intensity when you move. Is it better or worse, or the same? Maybe not all the information will be addressed, but it all matters because your body is relaying valuable information to you.
- Continue to scan your body, including your emotions, mind, heart, lungs, guts, bones, and your immune and nervous systems. How have your bowels been? Any symptoms from the gut are essential to note. The gut contains 500 million neurons, second to the brain's 100 billion neurons, and is considered the second brain. If you experience stress, it often appears as a symptom in the gut as well.[1]

- To focus on your immune system, think about how often you catch colds or viral infections, along with how severe they are. More frequent illness might indicate a weakened immune system. Also, assess the severity and frequency of your allergic reactions, whether they are seasonal, food-related, or skin reactions, since persistent allergies can indicate immune system overactivity or sensitivity. Additionally, be mindful of any chronic or recurrent infections, such as sinusitis or bronchitis, as these can be red flags for immune health.

- Consider your skin, since it is a crucial part of your immune defense. Do you have any frequent or recurring skin problems like eczema, psoriasis, or skin infections? Pay attention to how quickly you heal from cuts, bruises, or infections, as slow healing can also be an indicator of immune system issues.

- Now evaluate your nervous system. Start by paying attention to how often you feel stressed or anxious. Nervous system distress can significantly impact immune system health, too, as chronic stress and anxiety weaken the immune response, making the body more susceptible to infections and illnesses. When the nervous system is overworked, it can compromise immune function. All systems are connected, so you can begin to see the importance of managing stress on your entire health. You can also monitor your nervous system by tracking the quality and quantity of your sleep. If you're struggling with falling asleep, staying asleep, or feeling rested, these can be signs of nervous system imbalances.

- Observe your mood and emotions. How has your mood been lately? Have you tended to have mood swings, irritability, or emotional numbness? I address describing your emotions in chapter 9, so go back and use that chapter to define what your thoughts and emotions are telling you.

- Have you experienced any other physical symptoms lately, such as headaches, muscle tension, digestive issues, or rapid heartbeat?

- Assess your energy levels throughout the day. Extreme fatigue or hyperactivity can be signals of imbalance. Additionally, evaluate your cognitive function by observing your ability to focus, remember things, and make decisions.

Describing What You Feel

Some symptoms, like pain, can be notoriously vague and difficult to describe. However, using specific, descriptive language can help you better understand and communicate what you're feeling. For example, after my double knee replacement surgery, I felt a tense, unsettling sensation along my spine, almost like a warning that something was about to go wrong. Compare that to simply saying, "I have discomfort in my spine." Can you see the difference? By describing my symptoms in detail, my doctors were able to discern whether the issue was muscular or related to my nervous system. This kind of specificity not only helps you connect with your body but also provides essential clues for your healthcare team to pinpoint the source of the pain or discomfort.

Descriptive words can help bring clarity to our health symptoms, so I've developed a list of descriptive words to use or prompt new words that best match your concerns (see table 10.1). Start by picking one or two that fit your situation. Then, take it a step further if you want by using metaphors to bring your experience to life. For example, instead of saying, "My leg hurts in the morning," you could describe it as, "I feel a warm and tingly sensation that radiates from my kneecap outward to the back of my leg in the morning, like warm water pouring over my knee and dripping to the back."

This process is actually fun—you get to really "hear" what your body

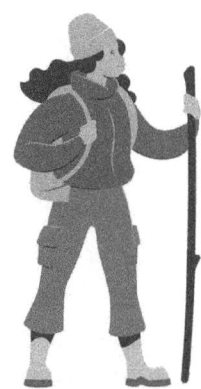

You can't solve what you can't clearly define.

is saying. Going through this process helps you spend time with your health status and understand it. Otherwise, it's hard to solve what you can't clearly define or describe.

Aching	Cramping	Gnawing	Heavy	Hot	Burning
Drilling	Itching	Crushing	Dull	Mild	Pulsing
Knotting	Locked	Deep	Superficial	Grabbing	Rubbing
Pinching	Stinging	Unsettling	Stiff	Tight	Unnatural
Prickly	Nagging	Taut	Piercing	Penetrating	Squeezing
Rasping	Consistent	Tearing	Continual	Thumping	Popping
Sharp	Shooting	Stabbing	Floating	Throbbing	Exhausting
Tingling	Pins and needles	Intense	Shocking	Spasming	Fluttering
Disturbed	Depressed	Unbalanced	Worried	Different	Atypical
Loose	Grinding	Sensitive	Flaring	Nervous	Pressure
Tense	Weary	Weighted	Chapped	Raised	Sore
Tender	Panging	Inflamed	Waving	Twinging	Straining
Intermittent	Radiating	Flashing	Pounding	Irregular	Pressing
Shaky	Looming	Pulsing	Mellow	Punching	Grasping
Foreboding	Pressure	Reoccurring	Racing	Subtle	Deep

Table 10.1: Descriptive Words for Pain and Discomfort

Descriptive words help pinpoint the exact nature of your sensations. For instance, instead of feeling a vague sense of unease, you might describe it as a "fluttering in the stomach" or a "racing heart." The more precise you are when communicating with your healthcare team, the better they can understand and address your concerns. It will also help you find interventions that are tailored to your symptom. You'll also be able to notice smaller, incremental improvements. And don't stop there—use these specific terms in your online research to narrow down your results and gain targeted and tailored insights.

The Big Picture: What Is Your REAL Overall Health Status?

We can get so focused on a particular ache or pain that it dominates the overall impression of our health. For instance, before I had my knee joints replaced, the pain made me feel like my health was in steep decline. It skewed my perception, making me feel far worse than I truly was. Yes, my knees were impacting my health, but they weren't the whole story. At the time, though, it certainly felt that way.

As I mention earlier, it's easy to misjudge our health—sometimes, we think we're in better shape than we are, or other times, we underestimate our health when it's actually better than we think. To help ground our health assessment in reality, I developed the Health Spectrum Pyramid (see figure 10.1). This tool helps you categorize your health into four levels, providing a clearer view of where you are, where you've been, and where you could aim to be.

Health Spectrum Pyramid

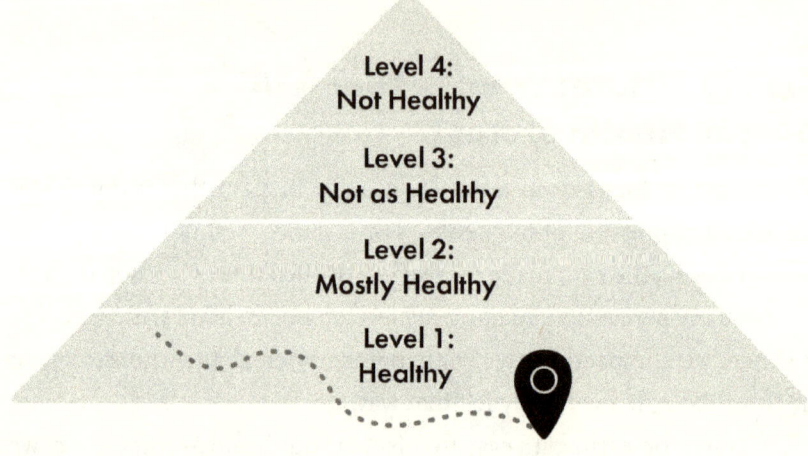

Figure 10.1: The Health Spectrum Pyramid

- **Level 1: Healthy**—You feel great with few health concerns. Though you may still get sick or injured occasionally, your health doesn't limit your lifestyle, and you feel well most of the time.
- **Level 2: Mostly healthy**—You generally feel good, but there are a few symptoms or issues that mildly restrict your life. You can live the life you want most of the time, but your health occasionally interferes with your activities.
- **Level 3: Not as healthy**—While you feel good sometimes, your health issues or symptoms are frequent and interfere with daily life. Medical interventions are becoming more routine.

- **Level 4: Not healthy**—You don't feel well most of the time. You may be managing a chronic or advanced condition that requires regular medical care. Your health limits your lifestyle, and those around you are concerned about your well-being.

This pyramid intentionally uses general terminology because health is subjective—we all perceive it differently. The goal is to help you assess your health honestly, from your own perspective.

Using the Health Spectrum Pyramid

Assessing where you fall on the pyramid only takes a few minutes and requires tuning in to your body. Here's how to apply it:

First, ask yourself: Where do I fall on the Health Spectrum Pyramid? Am I at Level 1, 2, 3, or 4? Once you have a general sense, back it up with reasoning by answering these questions:

- Are your symptoms interfering with your daily life? For how long?
- How many major health issues do you have?
- Are you currently on any medications?
- Do you visit the doctor frequently?
- Are your symptoms transient, or do they persist throughout the day or night?
- How many minor symptoms do you experience?
- How difficult would it be to improve your symptoms?

After reflecting on these questions, revisit the Health Spectrum Pyramid. Has your level shifted based on this new perspective?

> ## Monitoring Your Own Health
>
> Being in tune with our health and noticing aches and pains early allow us to quickly pick up on changes and recognize when something's off. As I discuss in chapter 16, it's important to track your efforts when addressing a health concern. Pay attention to even the smallest improvements and watch for positive trends over time. If you don't notice any progress, give it time—typically six to ten weeks—to fully assess whether your approach is working. If it's not, then try something different and monitor the results for another six weeks.
>
> By giving our interventions a fair chance—not just a week or two, but at least six weeks—we can better evaluate their effectiveness. This methodical approach helps us make informed decisions about our health. While this is a solid practice for most major health concerns, always take into account your unique circumstances.

What Now? Tailoring Interventions to Your Level

Now that you have a clearer sense of where you are on the Health Spectrum Pyramid, it's time to focus on the right interventions to move forward. While Level 1: Healthy may not always be attainable for some of us, aiming for a healthier level is still a fantastic goal. It's about meeting yourself where you are and working toward improvement.

In the coming chapters, we explore how to match your current Health Spectrum Pyramid level to appropriate intervention options. For now, here's a quick breakdown (summarized in table 10.2):

Level 1: Healthy

Celebrate! You should focus on maintaining your health with minimal medical interventions, concentrating on nutrition, regular activity, and mental well-being—what I call "building your health savings account." The more you invest now, the longer you'll stay in this optimal state.

Level 2: Mostly Healthy

Like Kristen, you're in a good position. Lifestyle interventions will help you maintain your wellness, while medical care can serve as prevention or maintenance. Complementary practices like massage, reflexology, or meditation can also reduce stress and prevent regression.

Level 3: Not as Healthy

If you're entering this level, focusing on lifestyle changes, complementary practices, and medical interventions can help you bounce back. But if you've been here for a while, more consistent efforts will be needed to see improvement.

Level 4: Not Healthy

At this stage, medical care becomes your primary focus, but lifestyle changes and complementary therapies can still support your recovery. Collaborate with your medical team to find treatments that align with your health goals.

HEALTH LEVEL	DESCRIPTION	FOCUS
Level 1: Healthy	Minimal medical intervention is needed. Focus on maintaining health through good nutrition, activity, and mental well-being.	Maximize health; build your "health savings account."
Level 2: Mostly healthy	Well-being is maintained with lifestyle interventions. Medical care is for preventive maintenance and occasional concerns.	Explore new ways to maintain health and build relationships with healthcare providers.
Level 3: Not as healthy	Health has declined, requiring more focus on lifestyle and complementary interventions, with regular medical care likely needed.	Commit to lifestyle changes and establish complementary providers (see chapter 15) to improve health.
Level 4: Not healthy	Medical care is the primary focus. Complementary therapies support symptom management and recovery alongside medical interventions.	Work closely with your medical team and incorporate complementary therapies to enhance recovery and lifestyle interventions (see chapters 14 and 15).

Table 10.2: Expectations for Each Health Level

Understanding your health status with clarity is nearly impossible without the right perspective. The Health Spectrum Pyramid offers an objective view, helping you avoid overreactions to minor issues or underestimating your needs when health declines. By using this framework, you'll be equipped to make informed decisions and guide your health with intention.

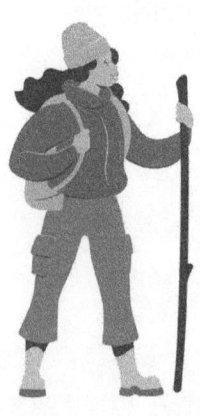

We can't chart a path to better health without first understanding where we stand.

True healing starts with knowing where you stand. From here, you can shift from reacting to your symptoms to strategically managing your health. This clarity empowers you to make choices that not only address your current health but also pave the way for consistent health management.

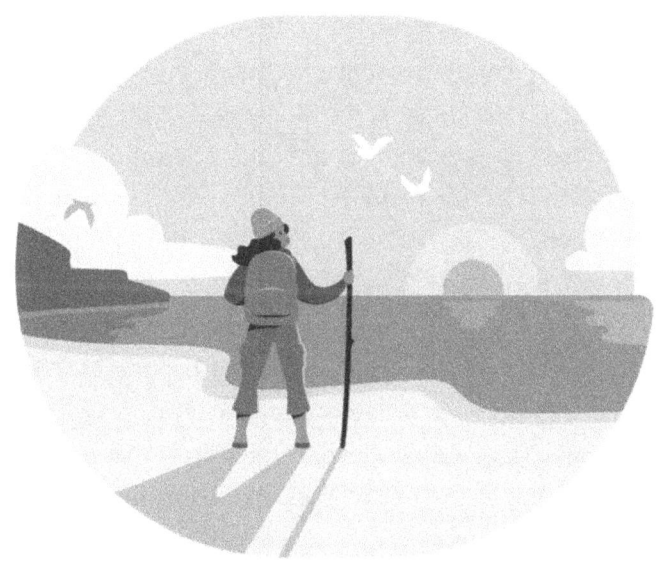

CHAPTER 11

CREECS: Defining Your Health Approach (The Six Questions Everyone Should Answer Before Making Any Health Decision)

Naturally, our desire to recover from illness or to improve our health and appearance is strong. So, when we do make health decisions, especially important ones, we often operate in a mode of anxiousness or fear. We long for the way we were and fear what will happen to us now that we have this health ailment. These two motivators are dangerous alone, and even more so together, because they can drive us to make hasty, uncalculated health decisions. That's why I want you to manage your emotions using information in chapter 9. But add to our escalated emotions enticing, seemingly easy health fixes, and we're vulnerable to making some really poor health decisions.

A good example of our desire for a quick and easy fix is the use of new drugs for weight loss. One study shows that 1 in 8 people have used medication such as Wegovy (also called Ozempic when used to control diabetes) for weight loss.[1] If you haven't tried it, you likely know someone who has. These drugs, called glucagon-like peptide-1s (GLP-1s) are found to be highly effective, with an average weight loss of 15 percent to 20 percent.[2] However, when stopped, studies show that people gain an average of 7 percent of the weight back, and some have lingering side effects, like a ravenous appetite.[3] GLP-1s cost around $1,000 a month and come with side effects, including muscle mass loss. The long-term side effects are still unknown.

Knowing this, would you try this medication? It all depends on your emotions (which you've already checked), values, preferences, and risk tolerances, and in order to know what those are, we need to ask ourselves some questions.

In the remaining chapters of this book, I talk about a lot of options you have for being healthy and healing your body. Before going there, however, this chapter challenges you to answer six questions we should all ask ourselves *before* putting together a health plan or making a health decision, especially a major one. Answering these questions will help you be confident in the decisions you make, and you will have your eyes wide open when you try health interventions. This will keep you from impulsive decision-making by giving you a realistic viewpoint of your health decisions. Here are the six questions.

The Six Key Questions

Before you commit to the surgery, procedure, medication, or supplement, ask yourself these six questions:

- How **committed** am I to this effort?
- How much **risk** am I willing to take with this intervention?
- How **effective** does this intervention need to be for me to feel confident in trying it?
- How much **effort** am I willing to put into this intervention and its recovery?
- What is the budget or **cost** threshold I'm willing to spend for this intervention?
- What kind of **support** or guidance do I need to do this intervention, and do I have that available?

I refer to these valuable six questions as **CREECS**: commitment, risk, effectiveness, effort, cost, and support. These questions reveal our unspoken preferences and needs and can help us discover health interventions that align with our preference parameters more quickly. You can even add questions to these basic ones—don't ever stop asking yourself what you value, how much you're willing to tolerate, etc. By asking questions, you begin to gain clarity in your limits. This will save you time and resources and draw you to the options that you feel are within your personal zone.

When you're left with a big health decision, spend some time asking questions about not only the options, but of yourself—what your limits are. Then, spend much of the other half researching for solutions and options that fall within your limits. Doing it this way will save you much time that would have been spent on looking for options that don't fit or suit you. Then, use the remaining time to go think through your decisions (using the information in chapters 6 and 7) so that you are confident with your final decision. The bigger the decision, the more time you should take thinking about what to do.

Let's dive into the six questions in more detail. Note that some of these questions may not apply to your current condition or health decision, so skip past those that don't apply.

C REECS Question 1: How committed am I?

How dedicated, consistent, and persistent are you willing to be over the long haul, even in the throes of setbacks? Look through these questions and honestly answer them, if they are applicable. Add your current condition into the question to make it personal.

- How important is resolving my health issue, (insert your issue here), to me?
- Am I prepared to make significant lifestyle changes, if needed? (Note: medical interventions often come with lifestyle modifications, so don't omit those from your overall consideration.)
- Is the commitment needed for this treatment or intervention something I see myself following through on over the long term?
- Am I willing to embark on a full course of recommended treatment, or does a more gradual approach suit me better?
- How committed am I to finding and treating the root cause of my health issue?
- Am I willing to go through the necessary recovery to receive the potential benefit?
- What would happen if I did not do this intervention I'm considering?

What did you find out about how much you're willing to commit to overcoming your health concern or intervention? Was it generally low, medium, or high? Make a note on some paper, saying something like this: "For this health issue or intervention, I lean toward a (low, medium, or high) level of commitment." The answer to this question will help you find an intervention that matches your commitment level. Then continue to learn about your risk comfort levels.

CREECS Question 2: What level of risk am I comfortable with?

Are you a risk-taker, or are you one to proceed cautiously when it comes to embarking on a treatment or health improvement program? Answer these questions to find out:

- How willing am I to explore alternative treatments or therapies with limited scientific evidence, even if they seem promising?
- What level of risk am I comfortable with when it comes to potential side effects or adverse reactions from a health intervention?
- Am I open to trying therapies or treatments with known risks if the potential benefits align with my health goals?
- How much risk am I willing to take regarding the financial cost of certain health interventions?
- To what extent do I value traditional medical approaches with established safety records over less conventional methods?

What did you discover about how much risk you're willing to take when trying health interventions to help your health concern or improve your health? Make a note, saying something like this: "When it comes to health interventions, I typically prefer to keep risks at (low, medium, or high) levels." Continue to find out how important effectiveness is to you when you try health interventions.

CREECS **Question 3: How effective does the intervention need to be?**

Do you prefer to tackle your health issue with one powerful weapon, or are you willing to use an arsenal of weapons to improve your condition over a more extended period? In other words, how effective should your interventions be, in your opinion? These questions will give you insight into the answer:

- How important is it to me that this intervention effectively improves my health concern?
- Am I looking for immediate improvements, or am I comfortable with gradual progress over time?
- Do I prefer interventions with a proven track record, even if they may come with more effort or cost?
- Would I prioritize an intervention's effectiveness over other factors, like convenience or minimal side effects?
- Is achieving the best possible health outcome the top priority for me, even if it means dedicating more time and resources?
- Am I more willing to try new-but-promising interventions or tried-and-true approaches?

What did you learn about your preferred approach to addressing your health concerns? Make a note of it, saying something like this: "Generally, intervention effectiveness is of (low, medium, or high) relevance to me."

Now, continue to discover how much effort you're willing to invest in trying an intervention.

CREECS Question 4: How much effort am I willing to invest?

Are you willing to put a large, medium, or small amount of physical and mental energy into your intervention? Answer these questions to find out:

- How motivated am I to engage in daily practices or routines that require time and effort to manage my health issue?
- What level of dedication am I willing to commit to when it comes to lifestyle changes, such as dietary modifications or regular exercise, to address my concern?
- Am I open to investing time and effort into complementary therapies or treatments, such as acupuncture or massage, even if they require consistent sessions or practice?
- How willing am I to adapt my daily schedule or activities to accommodate interventions that could help manage my issue?
- To what extent am I ready to explore and research various interventions to find the most effective and effort-efficient options for addressing my concern?

So, what did you find out? How much effort are you willing to give when it comes to dealing with your health issues? Take note, saying something like this: "I typically find myself ready to invest (low, medium, or high) effort in my health intervention."

Now, continue to learn about how important cost is to you when choosing an intervention.

CREECS Question 5: What is the cost I am willing to pay?

How much are you willing to spend on your health efforts for a particular intervention or treatment? Here are some questions to ask yourself:

- How much am I willing to invest in my health to address this concern effectively?
- Do I prioritize cost over effectiveness? Or am I willing to spend whatever it takes?
- Am I comfortable with allocating a significant portion of my budget to an intervention if it promises superior results?
- Would I explore interventions with higher costs if they are associated with reduced risk or faster recovery?
- Is the overall cost of an intervention a critical factor for me, or am I primarily concerned with achieving the best health outcome?

What did you find out about how important cost of interventions is in addressing your health concerns? Make a note like this: "Health intervention cost is a (low, medium, or high) priority for me."

CREEC**S** Question 6: What kind of support do I need?

How important or needed will support be once you make this health decision you're about to make? And what kind of support will it be—mental, physical, or financial? Consider support from healthcare professionals, family, friends, or even social communities—put them all out there for consideration.

I recommend you also consider your personal preferences when asking for help. Which of the three levels resonates most with you?

- Low (1): You can handle what's next on your own and don't need a significant support system. Or perhaps you're self-reliant and prefer to manage your health mostly on your own.
- Medium (2): You recognize the importance of having a support system but also prefer to have some level of independence. You're

open and willing to seek help and guidance, when necessary, but you don't require extensive support.
- High (3): You realize that you'll need a robust support system in place. You will need to actively seek guidance, emotional support, and assistance from healthcare professionals, family, friends, or other support communities.

Whichever default tendency you fall into, you are aware of the support you may need to find, if any. Here are some additional questions to think about:

- Am I comfortable researching and managing my health decisions independently, or do I prefer to have assistance and guidance from others?
- Do I already have a reliable support network, including healthcare professionals, family, friends, or sources, that I can turn to, or will I need to seek these out beforehand?
- Would I prefer to be part of a community or group that shares similar health concerns and goals to help me stay motivated and accountable?
- Do I feel more confident and motivated when I have someone to share my health journey with, or am I more self-reliant in managing my health?

How important is support to you when addressing your health concerns, in general? Make a note and create a summary, something like this: "I expect I'll need a (low, moderate, high) level of support through this health intervention."

Support is essential to any health strategy, and it goes beyond just having someone there physically. **Physical support** might include help with daily tasks or transportation to appointments, but equally important is **emotional support,** where encouragement and understanding from loved ones or support groups can make all the difference. **Social support**—connecting with others who share your goals—boosts motivation and accountability, while **professional support** from doctors, therapists, and other experts ensures you get the right guidance. Don't forget **financial support,** as being able to afford treatments or healthy lifestyle changes is crucial. **Structural support** involves having a work and home environment that allows you to pursue your health goals, and **informational** support provides the knowledge and resources you need to make informed decisions. Finally, **advocacy support** includes those who fight in your corner, helping you navigate challenges and stay on track. Without a strong network of these various types of support, the journey to better health can be exhausting and, at times, impossible. Whether it's making dietary changes, attending regular treatments, or exploring new therapies like acupuncture, having a well-rounded support system is key to success.

Too often the kinds of support I describe don't appear on their own—we have to seek them out. This can involve reaching out to healthcare professionals, family, friends, experts, or support groups who can offer guidance and encouragement. The effort you put into finding and building this network is worthwhile, as it truly takes a village to achieve our best health.

You don't have to wait until you have a health condition to build your support. You can start building your support team even now. For example, you can find health professionals that resonate with you and that you can go to when you need health support. I have been establishing my professional health support team for years to help me through my health issues: a massage therapist who came to me after I had double knee replacement surgery to ease my aching back from sitting and lying down all day, an amazing physical therapist I could trust to help me recover as rapidly as possible, a therapist to help me through the stress of what felt like a health crisis, and a friend to vent to.

Build your financial support, too. You may want to consider a high-deductible health insurance plan and opening up a Health Savings

Account (HSA) or adding a Flexible Spending Account (FSA) to your existing health plan to save money for the times when you need to pay for extra medical expenses. Ask your employer's human resources professional about what is available through your employer.

Whatever support system you need for whatever issue you have, whether it's a social worker, a nurse who does home visits or gives recommendations over the phone, or a buddy who can bring groceries to you when you're not able to get out—these relationships become your recovery team. Don't hesitate to lean on others; together, you will heal faster and navigate the complexities of your health journey with greater ease and bounce-back.

CREECS helps you prioritize what matters most and factor it into your choices, leaving you with a health decision that's perfectly tailored to you!

Example of a Personal Health Approach

Once you've answered the six health approach questions, CREECS, you are now able to produce a personal health approach—a comprehensive reflection of your preferences, values, and readiness to take charge of your health decisions.

Let me give you a couple of examples of health identities from two of my former clients, Denise and Ellen. Here is the one Denise crafted after going through the exercise of answering the six questions:

"I generally have a medium level of commitment—I often lose momentum after a week or two—and put in high effort for health interventions. I'll drive far, find the right doctor, take a lot of time to look online for options,

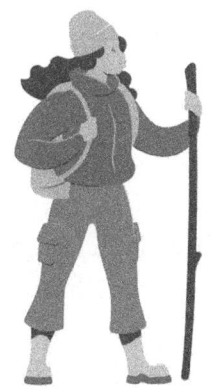

To safely navigate the tricky waters of health decisions, you must cross the CREECS first!

etc. I'm not afraid to have surgeries if needed, and I try different approaches. I want interventions with a high level of potential effectiveness and am comfortable with medium risk and cost when it comes to my health, but I will choose high cost if I think it's needed. I choose to manage my health independently, unless support seems beneficial. I don't have a lot of support in place so it would be a good idea to start building a support network."

When I asked Denise if anything she learned by answering the questions surprised her, she said, "I didn't realize my preferences for CREECS, so this is going to help me balance out my less helpful tendencies. I need to stick with an intervention instead of flake out. But I also shouldn't pick interventions that take too long, because I know I'll quit them. I can already see that I need accountability to get myself back in shape or I just won't do it, and that I like quick fixes. I'll go through the effort to find them, but I may not follow through. This is so helpful. Thank you!"

Another example, Ellen's personal health approach, is even more heartfelt and passionate than Denise's approach. Although she didn't follow the personal health approach template as closely as Denise did, what resulted was what feels like more of a personalized health mission statement.

"As a health adventurer and guardian of my well-being, I am dedicated and passionately committed to high-level effort and commitment to take care of my health. My desire to achieve my best health leads me to explore new interventions and health horizons. However, I am conservative when it comes to spending money on my health, and I seek value for every investment toward my health that I make. I am not afraid of taking moderate risks, although I do so with an educated and mindful approach because safety is of upmost priority to me. I am open to seek guidance and help, but I don't require or desire extra support unless it's necessary."

When I had Ellen create her personal health approach, she soon after began struggling with hip pain. After seeing her physician, she was told that hip joint replacement was necessary. Ellen took that information to heart, but because she had created her personal health approach prior, she knew first to try exercise, physical therapy, massage, and a therapy called dry needling, which didn't alleviate her pain. She was willing to spend money up front to be sure it was necessary to spend money on the hip replacement. Ellen educated herself on joint replacement apparatuses and was involved in picking which prosthetic she was going to use to replace her joint. Ellen called in some friends to temporarily help her recover. Ellen even asked me to come to her house to help her with post-surgery recovery exercises, knowing she would not have done them otherwise. That is an excellent example of the value of having a personal health approach!

What Is YOUR Personal Health Approach?

Now that you've identified your preferences, hold onto them firmly. Write them down and keep them close so that when you're faced with a major health decision, you can return to them as your guide. It's easy to lose sight of your preferences in moments of uncertainty or urgency, but the six CREECS preferences will ground you in who you are and what you value most.

By thoughtfully considering your level of commitment, risk tolerance, desired effectiveness, effort investment, budget, and support needs, you're not just making decisions—you're crafting a health approach that's deeply aligned with your personal values and goals. This preparation empowers you to manage your health intentionally, avoiding impulsive or random choices. With this foundation, you'll find the confidence to pursue interventions that resonate with you and the direction to follow through. Thoughtful preparation leads to better outcomes, and with your CREECS preferences in hand, you'll be ready to make decisions that truly reflect your unique path to health.

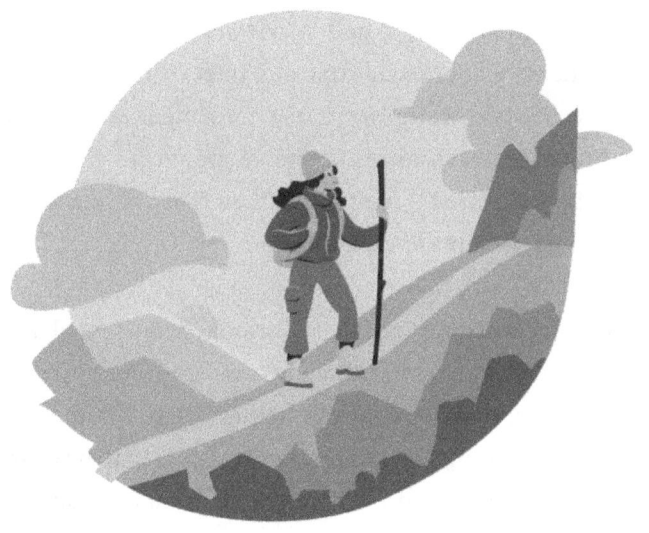

CHAPTER 12

Lifestyle Interventions, Part 1: The Core 4

In this chapter and the following three chapters, we explore and discover the potential of the three key approaches to health: lifestyle and complementary and medical interventions. These categories represent distinct yet interconnected pathways to healing and achieving optimal health. While most people are familiar with these, we often see them as separate options rather than pieces of a larger health puzzle. The truth is, each has its strengths and limitations, and understanding when to use each approach—or even better, how to combine them—can dramatically change the outcome of your health journey.

Typically, when we face a health challenge, we tend to focus on just a few potential solutions—those we've read about online, heard from a friend, or discussed with a doctor. We think that among these choices, there must be a good enough option. However, Health Heroes take a more comprehensive approach, exploring interventions from three distinct buckets: lifestyle, complementary, and medical. By broadening their view, they don't just find an acceptable approach—they uncover the *best one* for their situation. Then, these three types of interventions can be layered at the right time to maximize the impact on overall health and recovery. Let's start with lifestyle interventions.

Lifestyle interventions are often overlooked, dismissed as too slow or subtle to address serious health concerns. This misconception arises because these interventions typically require time for their effects to become visible. What many people fail to realize is that even small, positive changes can compound over time. For instance, a single glass of water can boost energy levels, or one nutrient-dense meal can stabilize blood sugar, but when done repeatedly, whole physiological systems work more optimally. When these habits are practiced consistently, they increase health resilience, resulting in a stronger defense against future health issues.

The challenge is that these changes, while powerful, aren't always immediately obvious. As a result, people assume they aren't impactful and abandon them prematurely when they don't see instant results. It's akin to expecting that a week of stretching will restore the flexibility of youth. We've all been there—losing motivation when improvements don't happen quickly. The problem isn't the lack of results but rather that our expectations are often misaligned with how lifestyle changes truly work. By understanding their cumulative power, we can set realistic expectations and stay committed to long-term health benefits.

There are dozens of lifestyle interventions to consider when creating a health plan, but four foundational interventions stand out, which I call the **Core 4**. These four—hydration, exercise, nutrition, and sleep—are essential to life. Without them, we cannot thrive. They form the foundation upon which all health is built. Before we explore other health intervention strategies in the later chapters, it's crucial to first address these areas, ensuring our bodies are properly nourished, active, rested, and hydrated. The Core 4 aren't just basic needs—they're the bedrock of health and the starting point for managing and optimizing our health. These are the nonnegotiables. No other intervention can truly succeed without them, no matter how advanced or promising. For example, imagine someone trying a cutting-edge supplement to boost their energy levels while neglecting their sleep. Despite taking the supplement, they're still exhausted because a fundamental physiological need—lack of proper rest—isn't being addressed. This oversight impedes their recovery and renders the supplement far less effective. Before exploring other options, this is where everyone should start. Master the Core 4 first, and you'll be setting yourself up for success in any other health endeavor you pursue.

Let's also examine the benefits of each component in more depth and understand why they are crucial to your physiological well-being.

1. Hydration

Water is the universal solvent. What does that mean? This means that water can dissolve more substances than any other liquid. And why is that important? Because water transports valuable chemicals, minerals, and nutrients while removing toxic elements that damage cells. It's highly efficient at this, but only if your system has enough water. Without sufficient water, you create a high concentration of toxins that the kidneys must filter. And kidneys need water to filter blood efficiently.

Daily, the kidneys filter about 1,800 liters of blood and excrete waste through urine around 300 times. So, if you're not hydrated, all your physiological systems suffer, down to every cell. This creates a toxic environment for your cells.

Water serves many critical functions in the body. It plays a key role in temperature regulation, acting as the body's natural cooling system. It aids in digestion and nutrient absorption, helping to break down food and ensuring that nutrients are effectively absorbed into the body. Proper hydration also supports joint lubrication, reducing friction between bones, improving joint movement, and increasing flexibility—so if your joints are aching, it might be a sign to drink more water. Additionally, water is essential for circulation, as blood is primarily water and is responsible for carrying oxygen and nutrients to cells while removing waste products. It also maintains electrolyte balance, which is crucial for proper nerve function, muscle contractions, and overall fluid balance. Last, skin health depends on adequate hydration, as water helps maintain skin elasticity, protects against external threats like viruses, and allows skin to function optimally—plus, hydrated skin often looks and feels better, which can even improve your mood.

Tips for Staying Hydrated

To stay properly hydrated, aim for about 75 percent of your daily liquid intake to come from water, with the remaining portion from other liquids. If plain water isn't appealing, try making it more enjoyable by adding slices of fruit, such as lemon or berries, or cucumber for a refreshing twist. Experiment with different flavors to make drinking water something you look forward to.

If you often forget to drink water, try making it more accessible. Keep a water bottle at your desk, in your car, or anywhere you're likely to spend time. The easier it is to reach for, the more likely you are to drink regularly throughout the day.

A simple yet effective tip is to drink a glass of water after every bathroom break. This routine ensures you're consistently hydrating without overthinking it.

If you're sweating heavily due to exercise, spending time in the heat, or if you're pregnant, increase your water intake to meet your body's elevated needs. The bathroom trick can also help compensate for these higher demands, ensuring you stay adequately hydrated. You'll quickly notice that increasing your water intake gets easier the more you practice it.

> ### How Much Water Should I Drink Every Day?
>
> You've probably heard the recommendation that we should all drink about eight glasses (sixty-four ounces) of water a day. But a better rule of thumb is to **listen to your body**—drink when you're thirsty and ensure your urine is light yellow or clear, which is a good sign of proper hydration. Don't forget that foods with high water content, like fruits and vegetables, also contribute to your daily hydration. For example, I personally love eating watermelon in the summer—not only does it taste great and have lots of water, but it's also packed with vitamins and minerals, helping to keep me hydrated as if drinking a sports drink (which typically have sugar and additives that aren't healthy). If you're more active or out in a hot climate, you will need to drink more to stay adequately hydrated. If your pee is light, you're hydrating just right!

2. Exercise

As an exercise physiologist and personal trainer, I'm passionate about this topic. Your body was meant to move. Studies show that even walking 8,000 steps a day can significantly reduce the risk of premature death.[1]

But all kinds of exercise benefit your heart, lungs, weight, mental health, immune system, sleep, and so much more. Here's a brief overview of the exercises I recommend you do, and why.

Aerobic Exercise

Cardiovascular, or aerobic, exercise strengthens your heart, lungs, and circulatory system. It helps your body build small blood vessels that transport oxygen and nutrients while removing carbon dioxide and metabolic waste. This process boosts metabolism, burns calories, increases blood flow, and keeps blood vessels clear. In essence, aerobic exercise keeps your heart and lungs function efficiently, while giving your skin a healthy glow.

To gain the benefits, your heart rate needs to rise above its resting level. A simple test is if you're slightly out of breath and can't comfortably hold a conversation when walking. You can also use a perceived exertion scale from 1 to 10, with 1 being no-to-very-little effort and 10 being all-out maximum effort. You want to aim for the zone between 5–8. At this level, you'll feel the physical effects without overexertion. Lower effort (1–4) won't provide cardiovascular benefits, while extreme effort (9–10) risks injury and requires more recovery.

Start with doing ten minutes more than what you do today. Then, increase how much you do by ten minutes every other week until you are doing aerobic exercise for thirty to sixty minutes per session. Ideally, it is good to do cardiovascular exercise two to three times weekly. You can also mix shorter and longer sessions or alternate intensities within a workout. The goal is to *enjoy it*—whether walking, biking, swimming, or hiking; if you like it, your body will crave the activity over time.

I also recommend incorporating a variety of activities, commonly known as cross-training. Switching up your activity now and then prevents injury, keeps your brain engaged, and promotes balance and flexibility. Remember, if you don't regularly challenge specific muscles or your cardiovascular system, you'll gradually lose strength and endurance in those areas.

Strength Training Exercise

While cardiovascular exercise targets the heart and lungs, strength training is equally important. Without it, muscle mass naturally declines with age (a condition known as sarcopenia), making us weak, fragile, and less functional in daily tasks. Strength training combats this loss and also maintains bone density, reducing the risk of osteoporosis. Strong muscles mean strong bones.

Strength training also supports metabolic health. Muscle tissue helps regulate blood sugar and burns more calories than fat, even at rest. Building and maintaining muscle boosts calorie burn and aids in weight management.

When starting or maintaining a strength program, target the entire body—arms, legs, back, chest, and core. Perform eight to fifteen reps per exercise, gradually increasing weight or reps as you progress. If you're just starting, aim for one set and work up to two as your body adjusts. By the last rep, you should feel the effort without compromising form.

Commit to thirty minutes of strength training two to three times a week, with rest in between. If you need guidance, consider hiring a personal trainer or exploring free online resources. Make exercise enjoyable, whether through fun clothing, a beautiful environment, music, or a workout partner. Enjoyment is the key to staying motivated.

Balance, Stretching, Coordination

While strength and cardio are essential, balance, stretching, and coordination are equally vital for a well-rounded fitness routine. These elements improve movement quality, reduce injury risk, enhance cognitive function, and protect against cognitive decline.[2]

Balance exercises strengthen the brain-body connection, aiding stability and preventing falls. Simple practices like yoga, tai chi, or standing on one leg work your core muscles and improve body control. Stretching keeps muscles and ligaments flexible, reducing stiffness and injury. Regular stretching after workouts or throughout the day maintains range of motion, with extra focus on tight areas like hamstrings and shoulders.

Coordination is another way to improve your body-mind connection and enhance physical precision and agility, making daily tasks easier. Activities like ball sports, tennis, or even games like cornhole and ping pong improve hand-eye coordination and reaction times.

Exercise Options Review

Table 12.1 summarizes the main different kinds of exercise and common recommendations for how often you should engage in them. As you can see, many activities offer a combination of benefits that span across different exercise types, allowing you to get more efficient use of your time. For example, dancing is a fun and dynamic way to work on balance, coordination, aerobic fitness, and flexibility all at once. Similarly, activities like yoga can improve flexibility, strength, and balance, while also providing a calming, meditative effect. Swimming is another excellent example—it builds strength, enhances cardiovascular health, and improves flexibility, all while being gentle on the joints. By choosing exercises that address multiple fitness components, you can maximize your workout sessions and enjoy a well-rounded approach to your health and fitness.

EXERCISE TYPE	AREAS OF FOCUS	FREQUENCY	DURATION
Aerobic exercise	Heart and lungs	Most days	30–60 minutes, moderate to high intensity (can't hold a conversation), walking, running, biking, etc.
Strength exercise	Muscles and bones	3–5 times a week	30–60 minutes, all body parts, intensity for general wellness, 8–15 repetitions, 1–3 sets
Balance exercise	Brain-body communication and muscle strength	Daily	No limit on how much, walking on uneven surfaces, standing on one leg, yoga, using balance equipment like Bosu
Stretching	Muscles and ligaments	Daily	Include all body parts, as long as it takes
Coordination	Hand-eye coordination and movement efficiency	Regularly (several times a week)	Ball sports, tennis, games like cornhole, or any activity that requires hand-eye coordination or precise movement

Table 12.1: Summary of Recommended Exercises

Inspired to Move

Exercise isn't a burden—it's a blessing. I learned this firsthand when my knees began to fail me. My world became smaller as I could no longer run, hike, or swim without pain. After double knee replacement surgery, everything changed. I started hiking, biking, and lifting weights again. I feel so alive, free, and *blessed*!

That's when I realized that movement is sacred. It's not something to dread or avoid—it's something to nurture. Exercise isn't torture; it's freedom. It allows us to do what we love without limitations. When we embrace movement and pay attention to how our body responds, exercise transforms from a chore into a gift.

Think of movement in all its forms—your heart, lungs, muscles, and bones all need it. Rotate, stretch, walk, and change your pace. Notice how your body contributes to your stability and strength. Move in ways that break out of the rigid patterns of daily life.

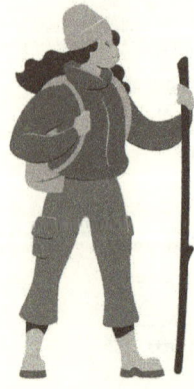

Exercise isn't a burden—it's a blessing.

We often fall into set routines, repeating the same motions until our joints stiffen and our range of motion shrinks. But when we shift our mindset from "I have to exercise" to "I want to move," we rediscover the joy in it. Movement becomes more than exercise—it becomes exploration, a way to push limits and expand possibilities.

Research overwhelmingly supports the benefits of regular exercise. It doesn't just add years to your life; it adds life to your years.

You have nothing to lose and everything to gain—start moving today!

What Exercise Is Best for You?

Deciding what exercise will work for you is all about listening to your body and trying to understand what it's telling you. Are you weak? Then strengthen it. Are you unsteady? Then practice balance. Are you stiff? Then stretch. Are you out of breath? Then get your heart and lungs in shape. Are you tired? Then rest. Get in tune with what your body needs, and over time, you will instinctively know how to exercise to keep it strong, flexible, balanced, and ready for anything. Building strength will come in handy when you face injury, illness, or nebulous health concerns because your baseline strength will be stronger and you'll have a greater capacity to recover. What do you have to lose?

3. Nutrition

Nutrition is one of the more personal aspects of Core 4. I find that people defend their way of eating like they defend their spending. It's a very touchy subject. But keep an open mind as we explore a new way to think about eating.

Don't think "diet," think eating smartly. Healthy eating is delicious, and it helps you feel amazing and protects your health. Plus, the social aspect of eating good food with others is therapeutic and good for us. Good nutrition also reduces the risk of diseases like diabetes, heart disease, and some cancers, and it's less complicated than you think. But Americans struggle to get the recommended nutrients for vitamins A, E, C, and zinc, among other nutrients.

To keep eating healthfully simple, think of managing your nutrition in the following three ways:

1. **Food Quality**
   - Food is more than just fuel; it has the power to heal. As Hippocrates famously said, "Let food be thy medicine, and medicine thy food." The nutrients in whole, natural foods directly affect your cells, promoting healing and resilience—or, if poor in quality, contributing to dysfunction. Foods straight from the earth, such as fruits, vegetables, legumes, and grains, are rich in these essential nutrients. Unfortunately, we've come to demonize some foods, like wheat, due to processing. But even refined grains have natural, minimally processed varieties worth considering.
   - The key is to focus on foods that nourish rather than harm. Organic options may be beneficial, especially for foods you consume frequently or that are more likely to be heavily treated with chemicals. Seek out unprocessed foods that retain more of their natural benefits.
   - Understanding food quality starts with curiosity. Read labels, research the nutrients in your food, and decide for yourself where you stand on topics like GMOs. It's not about obsessing over every

detail—just be mindful about what you put into your body. When you choose high-quality foods, you give your cells the best chance to build resilience, recover faster, and keep you healthy.

2. **Food Quantity**
   - The amount of food you eat plays a critical role in your health, and it's all about finding the right balance for your body. Ideally, your energy intake should align with your activity level. When you're recovering from an illness or injury, your body needs extra energy and nutrients to heal, so your intake should support that process. On the flip side, if weight loss is your goal, creating a modest daily deficit of 400–700 calories—through a combination of exercise and mindful eating—can lead to a steady, healthy weight loss of one to two pounds per week.
   - It's important to recognize that both overeating and undereating can have negative effects. Our bodies have ways of letting us know when we've gone too far in either direction. Feeling bloated, sluggish, or overly full after meals are signs that you may need to adjust your portions. If you occasionally overindulge, it's okay—balance things out by eating less at your next meal. The key is maintaining balance over time, not striving for perfection.
   - By listening to your body and being mindful of portion sizes, you can use food to support your health, particularly in maintaining a healthy weight. It's about tuning in to what your body needs and responding accordingly.

3. **Food Timing**
   - What and when you eat are both important factors in maintaining optimal health. The timing of your meals, the quantity of food throughout the day, and the types of nutrients you consume at certain times can all affect how your body processes food. Some people find success with intermittent fasting, when they limit their eating window to eight hours or less. While this

approach can be effective for some, it's not for everyone and depends on individual health needs and goals.

- One crucial aspect of food timing is understanding how different macronutrients—fats, proteins, and carbohydrates—affect your body at different rates. Fats burn slowly over several hours, proteins are digested over one to two hours, and carbohydrates are metabolized more quickly, usually within an hour. This information can be especially helpful for those with blood sugar concerns. By combining proteins and fats with carbohydrates at meals, you can slow the digestion of carbs, helping to keep your blood sugar and energy levels stable throughout the day.
- Beyond nutrient timing, the frequency of meals also matters. Some people prefer to eat multiple small meals throughout the day, while others thrive on just one or two larger meals. There isn't a one-size-fits-all answer—what matters is how your body responds. If you maintain a healthy weight and feel good overall, your current approach is working. However, if you notice signs of imbalance—such as low energy, mood swings, or frequent illness—consider adjusting food quality, quantity, or timing. You may need to space your meals differently or adjust the balance of macronutrients to improve how your body functions.
- Ultimately, timing your food intake can be another powerful tool to improve your overall health. By paying attention to how different foods and meal patterns affect your energy and well-being, you can make smarter choices that support both short-term and long-term health goals.

Nutrition as a Powerful Tool

By focusing on these three areas, you can use nutrition as a powerful tool for health and recovery without overcomplicating the process. Within each of these realms—food quality, quantity, and timing—you can adjust your intake throughout your life to meet your evolving nutritional needs. For example, as you age, you might prioritize more nutrient-dense foods like leafy greens, berries, and lean proteins to support bone health and muscle maintenance. You may also reduce portion sizes or increase calcium to protect your bones. As metabolic needs change, food timing can also be adapted, such as shifting to smaller, more frequent meals. By being flexible and mindful of these factors, you can ensure your nutrition supports your health at every stage of life.

Manipulating your food intake through food quality, quantity, and timing will give you plenty of options to find and adopt an approach that works perfectly for you. With this approach, no strict diet is necessary to manage your health. Instead of relying on rigid diets that often lead to frustration or burnout, you can make gradual adjustments that promote long-term health and healing. This flexibility allows you to enjoy food, maintain balance, and feel your best without the need for restrictive programs.

Good vs. Bad Food and Supplements

Another thing to note about nutrition is that you will come across claims about single foods or supplements being beneficial for specific ailments. Not long ago, acai berries were the buzz due to their high antioxidant content and were marketed as a superfood for heart health, weight loss, and antiaging. Over time, the excitement faded, just as it has with other superfoods. Today's focus is on mushrooms and fermented foods.

While superfoods like these have nutritional benefits, no one food is a miracle cure. As with most health trends, the claims around superfoods are often exaggerated. Foods don't work in isolation; they work together. The variety of foods you eat daily adds up to a complete nutritional picture. A single healthy food won't dramatically change your health, nor will avoiding one food. Instead, focus on eating a range of nutrient-dense foods to support faster healing and recovery.

Similarly, food deprivation is often misguided. Some diets avoid avocados because they're high in fat and calories, but avocados are rich in healthy fats, fiber, potassium, and vitamins. They're great for heart health and nutrient absorption. Bananas, often criticized for being high in sugar, are packed with potassium, vitamin C, and fiber. It's about balance, not avoidance.

Supplements can fill nutritional gaps, especially as we age. Supplements can be useful if you have specific needs, like supporting eye health. But many times, we're paying for supplements we don't need or that are too high in some nutrients or too low to make a difference in others. How do you know if this is the case? Do your homework. Read ingredient and nutrition labels. Add the nutrients from all of your supplements to determine if you're under or over the recommended allowance for each nutrient. Find books on the subject, talk to a registered dietitian, or do a deep dive online. Information is out there, waiting for you to find and apply it. Just be sure to go back to chapter 4 to make sure you're finding quality information.

If you're ready to take a supplement, look for supplements independently tested for quality, such as those with the USP Verified Mark, the NSF International symbol, or reviewed by ConsumerLab.com. These certifications ensure purity, potency, and safety. Also, look for the "U" symbol, which verifies that the supplement doesn't exceed the Tolerable Upper Intake Level (UL), which is the highest amount of a nutrient that can be safely consumed daily. Be careful if you shop for supplements at the vitamin store without doing homework. Once you find a supplement that fits the nutrient and safety criteria, consider the CREECS criteria mentioned in chapter 11. Make sure the cost is something you're willing to pay and that you're committed to the effort. Track results to assess if a supplement improved your health malady.

If you're unsure whether you have nutritional gaps, consider checking your blood levels for vitamins D and B12, iron, and other minerals. Personalized blood tests can also offer insights into where you might be deficient. You can also meet with a dietitian to get their perspective.

Additionally, logging your food intake for a few days using tools like MyFitnessPal or Cronometer can help identify any gaps in your diet. I do this every year to see where my diet might be lacking in nutrients, given my age. Where I see gaps in nutrients, I modify my food intake or supplement. In this way, you, too, can modify your nutrition to improve your overall health needs.

4. Sleep

Sleep is essential for physical repair, cognitive processing, and immune efficiency, reducing the risk of chronic illness and inflammation. A recent study found that those who slept less than six to eight hours per night had a 41 percent higher risk of cancer.[3] Sleep is important!

In *Why We Sleep*, Matthew Walker emphasizes sleep's role in memory, emotional regulation, and physical restoration, linking sleep deprivation to heart disease, diabetes, cancer, and cognitive decline.[4] He explains that consistent seven to eight hours of sleep each night improves longevity, cognitive function, and overall quality of life.

Good sleep also helps manage weight—those who sleep well are less likely to be overweight, while losing weight can improve sleep. To improve sleep, focus on hydration, exercise, and nutrition, and manage stress, optimize your sleep environment, avoid light before bed, and create a relaxing routine. Can you see how the Core 4 all intertwine?

Getting good sleep is no joke. Sleep has profound benefits for your physical health, mental well-being, and overall quality of life, making it worth the effort to improve your sleep habits. Prioritize sleep as a cornerstone of your health journey. Explore different sleep interventions and commit to trying them for at least six weeks to see what works best for you. If one approach doesn't improve your sleep, don't get discouraged—experiment with new strategies until you find what helps. Quality sleep is foundational to healing and overall well-being, so it's worth trying to refine your routine until you experience the benefits.

Working on Your Core (4)

Think of your health as a flowing river, with your body's innate ability to heal as the current. Each day, your cells are repairing damage while you sleep, and your hormones are orchestrating healing processes on a larger scale—directing your brain to process information, your immune system to repair and defend, and your liver and circulatory systems to break down nutrients for cellular use. Meanwhile, your digestive and urinary systems are clearing waste, ensuring your cells operate in a clean environment.

When you actively engage in practices like exercise, eating nutrient-dense foods, staying hydrated, and prioritizing sleep, you strengthen this natural healing current. These intentional efforts enhance your health and help you recover faster.

In short, the Core 4—hydration, exercise, nutrition, and sleep—represent **the primary pillars of health** and are the foundation of your healing journey (see figure 12.1). While other health behaviors like stress management and spiritual well-being are essential for a fulfilling life, these four elements are the most basic physiological needs. Your health will deteriorate without them, just as a table doesn't function without its legs. Next, let's explore other lifestyle interventions that further support your healing efforts and overall health.

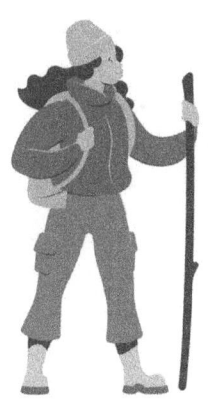

Think of the Core 4 as the four legs supporting a table. Remove a leg, and the table will become unstable. Remove two and good luck to you.

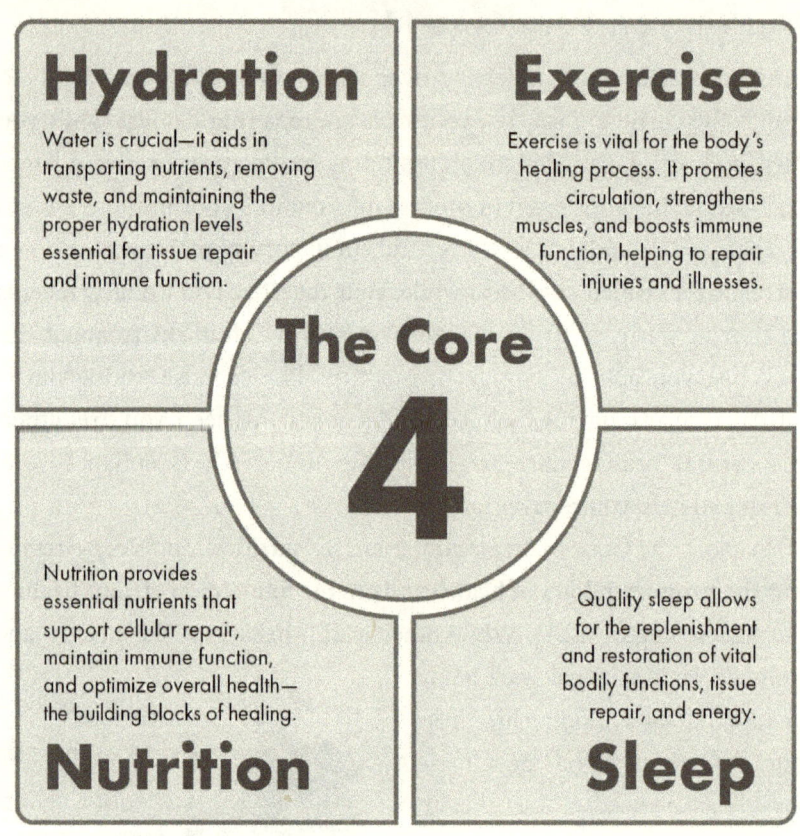

Figure 12.1: The Core 4 Lifestyle Interventions

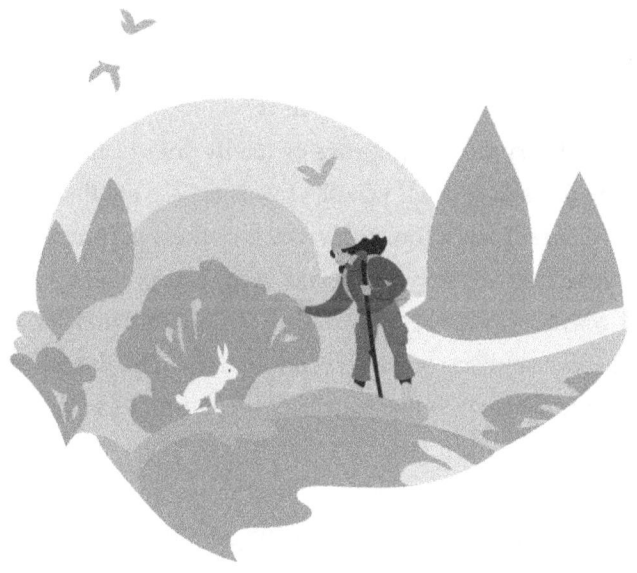

CHAPTER 13

Lifestyle Interventions, Part 2: Expanding Your Arsenal of Health Tools

The key aspect of a lifestyle intervention is that it is a self-practice or action you do **every day** to fortify your health. Making them daily practices is what makes them part of your lifestyle. Some lifestyle interventions hit the foundations of human needs, as in the Core 4 discussed in the previous chapter. But the others have other varying positive effectives on lives, in areas such as our desire to have relationships, health, peace, happiness, less stress, purpose, and meaning in our lives.

Although I could write an entire book about the vast realm of lifestyle interventions, in this chapter I compiled some of the most common options beyond the Core 4 to get you thinking about which might be good for you to try to help improve or fortify your health. As you look through the list, ask yourself what it is within your life that feels empty, neglected, or needs attention. Note which of these approaches strikes a chord in your heart as something you need. Is it peace? Or how about purpose? Maybe it's energy? Or maybe it's time to yourself? Take note and think about applying one intervention to try to fill the gap. Although one intervention may not flip your health condition around entirely or change your life, it just might.

What if you add a few new daily healthful practices into your daily life? Try practicing your faith and stretching in the morning (they can be done efficiently together), taking a meditative prayer walk in the afternoon, stating an encouraging mantra throughout the day, listening to positive music, and eating earlier in the evening. These simple (and free) self-practices will become habits, each building on the other so that after time you feel stronger during the day and sleep better at night.

Skeptics may think that doing small actions like these is a waste of time and energy, but that's far from the truth. They are the perfect way to fortify your mental, physical, and emotional health. I've seen my clients time and again move their health to a better health level by implementing a handful of lifestyle practices. Incrementally, you will make progress. But again, it may take a little time to see the impact, so be patient. Remember, it took your body time to get into the slump, so give it some time to get out of it.

I've put together a list of lifestyle practices for you to consider, but do some research and find your own. Use lifestyle interventions to fill the gaps in your life, cultivate better health, and get on the track to health!

From A to V: 18 Ideas for Lifestyle Interventions

To kickstart your thinking about lifestyle interventions that can enhance your life and your health, here's an overview of eighteen ideas, arranged in alphabetical order.

1. **Acupressure:** Apply pressure to specific points on your body to promote the flow of energy, healing, and circumvent pain.

2. **Aromatherapy:** Stimulate the sense of smell using aromatics and essential oils to induce feelings such as calm, alertness, and contentment.

3. **Attitude, joy, and happiness:** Develop the practice of peace, contentment, and happiness. That's right, it takes practice because we're naturally wired toward negative thinking (called negative bias).[1] Try practicing gratitude through journaling; find and read Bible scriptures that bring messages of faith, joy, hope, and peace; or read inspiring books. There are many ways to develop the attitude of joy and happiness. Whatever method you choose to use to build your positive attitude, joy, or happiness, there is research that shows that the practice of developing a positive emotional state can improve your overall health and spill over into improving other areas of living, such as sleep, relationships, and even financial success.[2]

> **Joy vs. Happiness**
>
> Note that joy and happiness are not the same. Knowing the difference can by itself produce peace. Joy is a deeper, more enduring feeling that comes from within and is related to inner peace and fulfillment. Happiness is a temporary state
>
> *continued*

> of pleasure or satisfaction that is often triggered by external circumstances. Both joy and happiness are important and valuable emotions, but understanding their differences can help you appreciate the deeper, more sustained nature of joy compared to the more transient nature of happiness.

4. **Biofeedback:** Use your mind to control your body by developing greater awareness of physiological responses through self-observation. This is a great way to manage stress, for example. First, become aware of how your body responds to the environment it's in. This is an excellent self-awareness skill. Then, practice calming your body using your mind during what your body perceives as stressful times.

- Monitoring devices such as heart rate monitors, pulse oximeters, or heart rhythm detectors can help identify specific physiologic responses to stress. With that information, you can choose a method to calm the nervous system using deep breathing. Most of us can control our heartbeat just by telling it to slow down, and we use that skill to regain composure and reduce stress. Visualization is another way people practice self-biofeedback—simply see yourself in a place of contentment, joy, and peace. This tells your body that there is no need to be alarmed.

- Biofeedback can be used to quit tobacco or handle difficult situations without getting upset. If this sounds interesting to you, do some research into an introduction to biofeedback to learn more. Biofeedback is a risk-free way to take control of your own physical and mental wellness.

5. **Environment:** Harmonizing inner energy with surroundings, such as in feng shui or decluttering, can create a sense of peace,

calm, and organization that results in reduced stress and feelings of anxiety. This can also include cleaning your immediate environment or removing contaminants and other health assaults.

6. **Exercise and movement:** One of the Core 4, this is so fundamental and important that there is a section dedicated to it in chapter 12.

7. **Faith, religion, and spirituality:** Reconnecting or strengthening your connection to a higher power to provide purpose and guidance can look different for everyone. However you choose to do this, it has been proven to reduce stress and anxiety and improve healing outcomes.[3]

8. **Hobbies:** Activities done for enjoyment or amusement can be a kind of health intervention. Art, crafts, building, writing, cooking, or mechanical work—whatever you choose, hobbies give the brain time away from perceived stress, resulting in improved mood.[4]

9. **Meditation, breathing, and mindfulness:** All these practices focus on resting and controlling the mind, emotions, and breathing. There are numerous variations of these techniques, all aimed at intentionally paying attention to thoughts or experiences. This mindfulness can enhance mental clarity, reduce stress, manage pain, and improve overall health.[5]

10. **Music therapy:** Listening to and playing music has shown to positively influence physical and mental health.[6] Just try listening to an angry song and assess your mood. Then listen to a positive song or peaceful music and do the same. Do you notice a difference? Music can shift our mood in just a few quick minutes.

11. **Nutrition and hydration:** These two are part of the Core 4 mentioned in chapter 12. If you haven't guessed by now, they are foundational, and that's why I can't state their importance in your overall health and well-being enough.

12. **Outdoor therapy:** From improving mood to increasing activity levels, nature nurtures us. Research shows that there are many

benefits to spending time outside. Getting outdoors for around fifteen to thirty minutes a few times a week can help your body produce enough vitamin D from sunlight, depending on factors like skin tone, geographical location, and time of year. Vitamin D plays a crucial role in our overall health, such as maintaining healthy bones and teeth, supporting immune and cardiovascular health, and regulating mood. Being outdoors also improves our balance, spatial awareness, visual acuity, hearing, and mental well-being. Exercising outdoors also adds the physical benefits as well.[7]

13. **Pets:** From snails to llamas, pets pack a powerful health boost. They can significantly improve our health by encouraging physical activity, facilitating outdoor time, and helping to manage loneliness and depression. The companionship they provide reduces feelings of isolation and boosts overall mood. Interacting with pets can lower blood pressure, reduce stress levels, and promote relaxation. Caring for a pet can also give you a sense of purpose and routine, which can be particularly beneficial for mental well-being. But not everyone is a pet lover, and pets do require time, effort, and financial resources for their care. Pets can be stressful, so having a pet is a personal decision that should be made based on your lifestyle, preferences, and ability to commit to the responsibilities associated with your animal companions.[8]

14. **Simplification and organization:** Similar to environmental interventions, organization as a lifestyle management technique can significantly improve our health by reducing stress, increasing productivity, and creating a harmonious living environment.[9] But organization can involve more than our environment around us; it also encompasses time management, financial organization, and even automation of tasks that we don't need to do. Think about washing dishes by hand versus using a dishwasher. That's a simple example, but when you start applying automation in areas such as bill paying, it can bring a great sense of relief and control.

15. **Sleep management:** One of the Core 4 mentioned in chapter 12, sleep produces growth hormones and other repairing hormones that generate new cells and repair tissue damage. Sleep also helps us process the information gained from a long day of wakeful living experiences. Sleep also stabilizes our emotions, so we wake up ready for whatever comes our way. If we don't get good sleep, our immune systems suffer and we get sick—so prioritize sleep as one of your go-to lifestyle interventions.

16. **Social interactions:** Quality human interactions and connections enhance mental well-being by reducing stress and feelings of loneliness, while also fostering a sense of belonging and support that can improve overall health and happiness. Social interactions have been found to improve immune function, too. Although socialization has been found to be beneficial for health, the amount needed varies from person to person. It's important to listen to your internal cues to determine the right balance of social interaction for you. Introverts, for example, may find that they don't need as much social engagement as extroverts and can feel content and energized with fewer interactions. Pay attention to how you feel after socializing—if you feel refreshed and uplifted, you might need more interaction; if you feel drained or overwhelmed, you might need less. It's all about finding what works best for your individual well-being. Trusting your internal signals and adjusting your social activities accordingly can help you maintain a healthy balance that supports your mental and emotional health.[10]

17. **Stress management:** Lifestyle and other strategies, such as progressive relaxation, guided imagery, and even humor, can help you overcome worry, stress, depression, and anxiety. The Core 4 found in chapter 12 all help reduce stress. Many other of the lifestyle interventions listed here also can reduce stress.[11]

18. **Volunteering:** Volunteering is simply serving others, and it is a powerful way to improve both mental and physical health while making

a positive impact on the community or in your family or immediate social circles. By reducing stress, enhancing mood, increasing physical activity, and fostering social connections, volunteering can help you feel healthier and more fulfilled.[12] Give a little, and you receive a lot of health in return.

Dietary Supplements, Herbs, and Essential Oils

As a culture, we often assume that our bodies need assistance in the form of supplements, a category that includes herbs and essential oils, so I would feel remiss if I didn't touch on this topic.

I mention supplements in the nutrition section in chapter 12, but I'm broadening this to include supplements beyond vitamins and minerals. Supplements of all sorts, from maca powder to astragalus and Stamets mushroom capsules, are another way to self-intervene when faced with a health issue or to support health. Taking a powder, elixir, oil, or pill to help our body is an intriguing and compelling practice—and it's easy. That's why many people practice this lifestyle intervention. Dietary supplementation is a $30 billion-plus industry.[13] A vitamin, mineral, amino acid, herb, or distilled oil from a plant are intended to support a physiological function, such as immune health, or address a specific health condition, such as sleep.

However, be alert to the fact that supplements are not well regulated, which is concerning. Many supplements don't contain what they say they contain in the quantities stated on the bottle. And most supplements are not rigorously tested as a prevention or treatment for conditions that they are promoting to address. One study found that 40 percent of fifty-seven supplements purchased online did not contain a detectable amount of the ingredient listed, and half contained the wrong amount.[14]

They also may contain contaminants, so look for some regulatory label, such as ConsumerLab.com, NSF International, and U.S. Pharmacopoeia (USP), so that you know your supplement was tested.

If want to take a supplement or use herbs or essential oils, I'd like you to think before you do and make sure you've considered all the angles. Supplements are sticky snares of promising benefits not often proven. Be wise by thinking twice before starting to spend your money on supplements. I've got some other tips so you can be sure that you're going in with eyes wide open and aware.

Tip 1: Call a professional. When it comes to taking supplements, it's essential to be both informed and cautious. While supplements can offer valuable health benefits, they can also interact with medications or other supplements in ways that aren't always obvious. This is why it's a good idea to run your supplement choices by a healthcare professional before you start taking them. A simple conversation with your pharmacist, doctor, or even a registered dietitian can help ensure that what you're adding to your routine is safe and beneficial. Pharmacists are particularly accessible—they can often provide quick advice, and many pharmacies have consultation services you can take advantage of at no cost. Checking for potential interactions is especially important if you're already on medications or other supplements.

You can also call your doctor's office and ask a nurse to pass the question along to your physician. This small step can prevent negative interactions and potentially save you money by steering you away from unnecessary or harmful supplements.

Registered herbalists are another resource to consider. While they have extensive knowledge of herbs and vitamins, it's important to remember that they may also want to sell you their products. That's not necessarily a bad thing—just be aware of the potential for bias. However, working with an herbalist does mean you're being monitored by someone with expertise, which can provide added peace of mind.

In short, consulting a professional before starting a new supplement is a wise move. It's a simple step that can make a big difference in ensuring your health is protected and your money is well spent.

Tip 2: Research the evidence. Look for solid information from the National Institutes of Health (NIH) Office of Dietary Supplements, or other reputable sources, to find scientifically backed resources to review the effectiveness of the supplement for your condition. Is the research limited, or promising?

Tip 3: Understand the supplement regulatory environment. Be aware that dietary supplements are not regulated by the FDA in the same way as medications. This means their safety, efficacy, and quality can vary widely. Look for supplements that have been tested by independent organizations like NSF International, U.S. Pharmacopoeia (USP), or ConsumerLab.com for quality assurance.

Tip 4: Be skeptical of claims. Be cautious of supplements that claim to be a "miracle cure" or "magic bullet." If it sounds too good to be true, it probably is. Understand that many supplement companies use persuasive marketing rather than scientific evidence to sell their products. Also, be leery of those touting the benefits of supplements. People usually mean well when they share their supplement stories, but your needs are unique, so graciously listen, but be skeptical.

Tip 5: Consider the cost-benefit ratio. Weigh the potential benefits of the supplement against its cost. Consider if the money spent on supplements could be better used on proven treatments or healthy lifestyle changes. Only consider supplements that have shown clear benefits for your condition and are recommended by trusted health professionals.

Tip 6: Consider a lifestyle before supplements. Focus on proven health strategies like a balanced diet, regular exercise, adequate sleep, and stress management before turning to supplements. Remember that supplements should complement, not replace, healthy lifestyle habits and conventional treatments. Also, be realistic in your expectations. A vitamin or supplement won't overturn poor health behaviors.

Tip 7: Track your progress. Keep a journal to record any changes in your symptoms, side effects, and overall health after starting the supplement. This can help you gauge its effectiveness. I help you do that in chapter 16.

While supplements can sometimes provide a beneficial boost, we frequently use them as a substitute for healthy lifestyle behaviors. This trade-off can be misleading, as many supplements may only offer a positive placebo effect at best. Before reaching for a supplement, ask yourself: Does my body truly need this? Or does it need rest, hydration, movement, and good food—the Core 4 essentials? These foundational elements of health are often more effective in supporting our well-being than any supplement could ever be. Prioritize the Core 4 to give your body what it truly needs to thrive.

Consider Journaling

Journaling is more than just writing—it's a powerful tool that can transform your health, unlock your creativity, and provide a therapeutic outlet all at once. I can't say enough about the benefits of journaling. Journaling can have numerous positive effects on your health, both mental and physical. Here are several ways in which journaling can contribute to overall well-being:

- **Stress reduction:** Writing about thoughts and feelings provides a healthy outlet for stress and emotions, which can reduce overall stress levels. Journaling can help you organize your thoughts and gain perspective on stressful situations, making them seem more manageable.
- **Improved mood:** Reflecting on positive experiences and accomplishments can enhance mood and promote a positive outlook on life. Keeping a gratitude journal—listing things you are thankful for—has been shown to improve overall happiness and emotional well-being.

- **Mental clarity and problem-solving:** Writing can help clarify thoughts and feelings, making it easier to understand them. By journaling about challenges, you can better identify solutions and strategies for overcoming obstacles.
- **Therapeutic effects:** Journaling can serve as a form of emotional release, helping to process trauma and negative experiences. It can help you explore your inner thoughts and feelings, leading to greater self-awareness and personal growth.
- **Physical health benefits:** Some studies suggest that expressive writing can improve immune function by reducing stress and promoting emotional well-being. For those with chronic conditions, journaling can help manage symptoms by providing a space to track symptoms, medication, and triggers. Writing about emotional experiences has also been shown to reduce the intensity of physical pain. Journaling before bed can also help clear the mind of racing thoughts, leading to improved sleep quality.
- **Cognitive benefits:** Writing things down can improve memory and comprehension, helping you to retain and understand information better. Regular journaling can also enhance cognitive functioning and critical thinking skills.
- **Creativity:** Journaling encourages creative expression and can stimulate creative thinking and problem-solving.
- **Practical benefits:** Journaling helps track progress toward goals and provides a record of accomplishments and milestones, as well as a great method to track interventions to see if they're benefiting you.
- **Motivation:** Writing down goals and tracking progress can increase motivation and accountability.

So grab a pen and let your thoughts flow—you never know what insights, ideas, or breakthroughs might be waiting on the page!

Which Lifestyle Interventions Belong in Your Personal Health Plan?

As I said, there are countless lifestyle interventions you can explore to enhance your overall health. From the Core 4, which again include regular exercise, balanced nutrition, hydration, and adequate sleep, to outdoor therapy and journaling, these strategies offer various ways to help you be your healthiest.

Try incorporating some of these interventions for at least six weeks and journal to see if they are effective. Be patient and give each one at least six weeks to show up positively in your health, and don't get discouraged if it seems that progress is slow. Trust me, these approaches are doing their work beneath the surface—down where the source of problems begin, like at the cellular level, within the tissues, or within physiological systems. Add one or two new lifestyle interventions to your routine for a minimum of six weeks and see what happens! Remember, it's about finding what fits your unique situation and finding what fits you the best.

In many cases, the more you do, the better you feel. Their positive effects can compound, resulting in faster healing. They also come with relatively low cost and risk. Sadly, many times these approaches are underestimated in their power to heal and keep us healthy. Take stretching, for example. This simple self-practice keeps our joints limber, thus preventing injury. Yet how many people stretch daily? Others produce more noticeable benefits. For example, regular exercise can significantly improve sleep quality, body weight, blood pressure, and stress levels. Reducing processed food intake can alleviate headaches, enhance mood, and promote gut health. Often, these simple changes can lead to profound improvements in overall well-being.

Another thing I love about lifestyle approaches is that by implementing them, you begin to learn more and more about your body and how it responds. When you start to introduce positive lifestyle behaviors into your day, you begin to see that your body is feeling different, your mood changes, or sleep improves. Your body does talk, so listen to what it's saying as you implement lifestyle interventions into your routine. Learn what it likes, doesn't like, and what it needs. This is the great experiment, and you are both the scientist and the subject.

Now that I've covered lifestyle interventions, there are two other intervention types to consider as you develop your own health plan: complementary and medical. I discuss these other two interventions in the next two chapters and then explore how to bring all three components together in your individualized health plan.

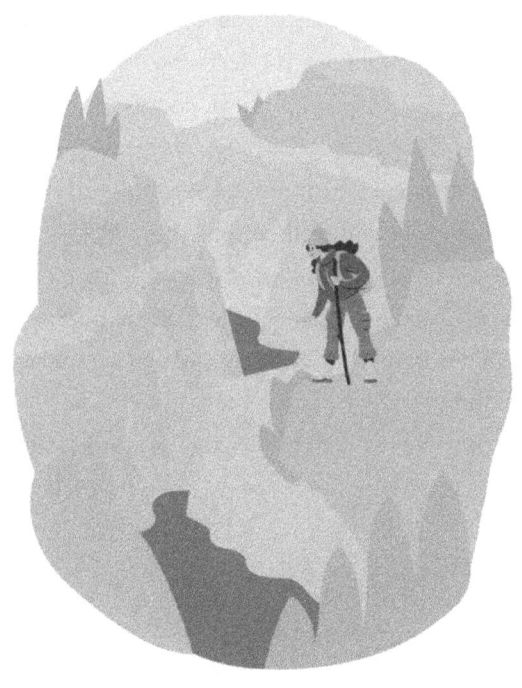

CHAPTER 14

Getting the Most from Conventional Medicine

For most people in the U.S., doctors are considered the gatekeepers to our best health. Modern Western medicine, also called allopathic or conventional medicine, is the go-to approach in the U.S. Research shows that a significant majority of Americans rely on conventional medicine as their first line of approach to managing health.[1] We heavily trust the highly educated and rigorously trained healthcare practitioners, including doctors, nurses, and pharmacists, who are armed with advanced degrees, vast clinical experience, and state licenses. These professionals are tightly regulated by federal and state authorities to ensure public safety. We trust the tests, prescribed medications, and recommended treatments. But should we always?

Most people find themselves within the medical-centered paradigm—they get tested, find their conditions, and treat them. For someone who expects this as the best outcome, this works fine. But some people do not want to be *treated*—they want to *heal*. And in many instances, there are no healing options discussed at the doctor's office because, as in the case of my asthma, there is no hope of healing in conventional medicine for many chronic conditions.

In this chapter I want to acknowledge the valuable contributions that conventional medicine makes to our health, discuss some limitations of this medicine, and help you find ways to get the most from conventional medicine.

Benefits and Challenges of Modern Medicine

Modern medicine excels in many ways—it's highly effective at treating acute conditions and keeping people with chronic diseases alive through advanced interventions. When it comes to emergencies, trauma, or clearly defined conditions, modern medicine acts as triage medicine, swiftly addressing the most urgent issues to stabilize and sustain life. As a consequence, modern Western medicine excels at saving lives, managing trauma and acute infections, dealing with medical and surgical emergencies, and identifying physiological abnormalities such as cancer. It also monitors progress when treating lingering issues.

However, putting all our faith in conventional medicine is not wise. When it comes to nebulous or complex conditions that don't fit neatly into diagnostic categories, modern medicine often struggles. These conditions may require a more holistic or integrative approach, something that triage medicine isn't always equipped to provide. While it can manage symptoms and prevent deterioration, it may not always get to the root cause or offer true healing for conditions that are less defined.

Here is an example: Thyroid dysregulation is one of the most common diseases worldwide. In the United States, it is estimated that 20 million people have some form of thyroid condition, and women are five to eight times more likely than men to have thyroid problems, with one in eight women developing a thyroid disorder during her lifetime.[2]

Often, hypothyroidism goes undiagnosed for a significant amount of time, which can put patients at risk for other medical complications. Many people have their thyroid removed because it stops regulating properly. Yet, many holistic approaches address thyroid disfunction as a condition that can be reregulated. Many times, dysregulation comes during or after disruptive life events, such as problems or stress with work, school, relationships, or money. And, by the way, if you are one of the 70 percent of Americans experiencing stress over money, you must address both your health issue and your financial health. If you address just your health and not your financial stress, the health issue will likely return, or another one will appear.[3]

A good personal example of how stress impacts health comes from the time my mom was told by her doctor to have her thyroid removed, which was exactly at the same time my dad was scheduled to go through laser knife surgery on his brain tumor. Was it a coincidence that my mom's thyroid became dysregulated at this stressful time? I don't think so—it's too coincidental. Could her thyroid have been reregulated? I believe it could have, but I don't know how long that might have taken and at what risk. However, if it were me, I would have at least investigated the possibility of keeping my thyroid and what might have been some options to try to reregulate my thyroid hormones.

Don't misunderstand me. I don't fault my mom for choosing to radioactively kill her thyroid (which left her unable to take care of my dad as he recovered from surgery because she was radioactive); I fault modern medicine. I also think we are forced to rush into a decision, so we pick the fastest, easiest (at the time) medical fix. In most cases, we can and should take time to investigate our options. Instead, we are rushed into decisions by the medical practitioners who are quick to bring the worst-case scenario to light if we were to wait much longer (many times without full regard to actual risk). Such is the way of conventional medicine.

Modern medicine can be highly effective, but it also comes with various challenging downsides. These include the following:

- **Cost:** Medical care can be expensive. High costs can lead to financial stress for patients.
- **Drug resistance:** The overuse of antibiotics and other medications has led to drug-resistant strains of diseases, making some treatments less effective over time.
- **Focus on treatment over prevention:** Modern medicine often prioritizes treatment over prevention. Preventive healthcare and lifestyle factors may receive less emphasis.
- **Fragmented care:** The modern medical system can be fragmented, with different specialists focusing on specific areas. This may lead to a lack of holistic care and coordination.
- **Invasive procedures:** Some medical interventions involve invasive procedures, which may be painful and carry certain risks. Surgery, for instance, can lead to complications.
- **Limited time with doctors:** Doctor-patient interactions are often limited in time, which can result in patients feeling rushed and not having their concerns fully addressed.
- **Misdiagnosis:** Medical conditions can sometimes be misdiagnosed, which can lead to unnecessary treatments or delays in receiving proper care.
- **Overreliance on medication:** In some cases, modern medicine may prioritize pharmaceutical solutions, leading to an

overreliance on medication when lifestyle and complementary approaches might be more appropriate.

- **Side effects:** Many medical treatments, especially medications, can have side effects that range from mild to severe. These side effects can sometimes outweigh the benefits of the treatment. Polypharmacy refers to the use of multiple medications by an individual. As the number of medications increases, side effects increase significantly.[4] This can range from mild effects like drowsiness or nausea to more severe complications. The risk of adverse drug reactions (ADRs), which can sometimes be serious or life threatening, also increases.
- **Stress and anxiety:** Medical tests and procedures can sometimes cause stress and anxiety in patients, which can have negative effects on their overall well-being.

While modern medicine has made remarkable advances and offers lifesaving treatments, as you know, it's not without its drawbacks. But a Health Hero knows when to leverage the strengths of modern medicine while being mindful of the potential downsides, ultimately aiming for the most effective and holistic approach to their health.

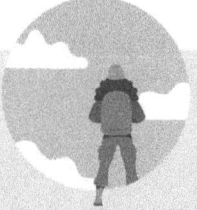

Q&A WITH ALICE: HEALTH INSURANCE

In the U.S., unlike in other countries, the question of physician visits always involves health insurance. I often get asked, "I don't have health insurance, and I can't afford to go to the doctor. What should I do?"

I understand how frustrating it can be to navigate the healthcare system without insurance. It can feel like you're stuck,

continued

especially when getting the care you need seems out of reach. The truth is, many of us, whether we have insurance or not, sometimes feel like we're at the mercy of an imperfect system. We wish healthcare worked better for everyone—where care was accessible and timely for all.

While the system may have its flaws, focusing on what you can control is key. Prioritizing your health through the Core 4—exercise, nutrition, sleep, and hydration—can make a big difference in keeping yourself healthy and potentially reducing the need for medical care. There are also many no-cost or low-cost lifestyle and complementary interventions available that can help you manage symptoms and support your overall well-being.

If you do face a medical emergency, remember that the healthcare system is still there to provide care when it's truly needed. In the meantime, take proactive steps to maintain your health and explore community resources, clinics, or programs that might offer medical support at a reduced cost or even for free. You're not alone in this—keep doing what you can to take care of yourself, and don't give up. Help is there; you will just have to find it.

Finding a Physician Who Fits You

When you find yourself in a position where traditional medicine is the best option, it's critical that you work with providers who are a good fit for you and your approach to making healthcare decisions. Finding such a healthcare provider can be challenging and often requires persistence and patience. The U.S. faces a healthcare provider shortage, making it difficult to find a doctor, especially one covered by your insurance or who is a good fit for your needs.⁵ This shortage can make it even more important to approach the process thoughtfully. Here are some tips to help you navigate this journey:

1. **Check with your insurance provider.** Start by contacting your insurance company to find in-network, high-quality doctors, whether you're seeking a specialist for a specific condition or a general provider. While general practitioners can offer broad care, they might not always be up to date on specialized needs. However, if you're up front about your specific requirements, they may refer you to a specialist who is. Don't hesitate to ask for referrals; many doctors are happy to connect patients with the right care.

2. **Ask for recommendations.** Reach out to friends, family, and colleagues for recommendations. Personal experiences can provide valuable insights into a doctor's bedside manner, effectiveness, and reliability.

3. **Consider virtual care.** If you're struggling to find someone locally, consider virtual care options. Telehealth services have expanded significantly and can provide convenient access to healthcare, especially in rural or underserved areas.

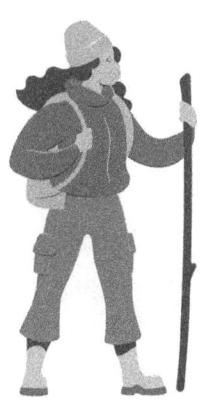

Remember, finding the right provider may not be easy, as doctors, like anyone else, have varying strengths and weaknesses. Aim to find a doctor who communicates well, empathizes with your situation, and has reasonable availability. While this may sound easier said than done, especially given the strain on the healthcare

Your doctor may know a lot about the human body, but they know little about the specifics of yours! It's up to you to fight for what will work best for you.

system, be patient. The system may not always be perfect or hospitable, but leverage its strength: treating conditions. Keep in mind that while the process may be frustrating at times, perseverance can lead to finding a provider who meets your needs.

Questions to Ask Yourself Before Seeing a Doctor

It is up to us to look at conventional treatments with a keen eye on what they can provide us to help us overcome our health challenges, and what they can't. We need to know what to expect from modern medicine, or it will become the go-to in all cases, even when it's not the best option. Ask yourself these questions when you're tempted to make a doctor's appointment: What am I expecting from this visit? If they tell me to take a medication or go through a procedure, what will I then do with that information? Is what the doctor recommended the only way to address my health problem?

We need to be prepared before we go to the doctor's office so that we are not pressured to do this or that just because they say so. We need a plan to make sure that what we do is logical, thoughtful, and aligns with our philosophical approach to health and healing. Keep in mind that medical interventions are always an option, but be willing to experiment with lifestyle and complementary interventions as well—keep them all in mind when visiting the doctor for advice and treatment.

Why is modern medicine so tricky? I believe it's because we think our health is broken when we're sick or injured and it needs to be fixed ASAP. We aren't patient with the healing process, or we've been so out of touch with our health status that we've let symptoms go unnoticed and they have progressed to more serious health issues. Then, we go to doctors mainly out of fear of a life-changing disease or illness. Often we find ourselves accepting a diagnosis and treatment when we shouldn't, or deciding to try to heal ourselves when we shouldn't.

The typical scenario goes like this: We meet with our doctor, they begin assessing our condition using various tests, and then they share their conclusions. Often they diagnose us with a condition, then offer a treatment to address it or help with the discomfort. Go to doctor, get tested, get diagnosed, get treated.

The better scenario would look like this: Meet with our doctor, they assess our health, and then they give their conclusions and potential treatment plan. We take that information and process it using a system (of which I've created for you and can be found in later chapters), and then we decide what is best after research and thought.

What's the difference? In scenario 1, we accept the doctor's answer as the best course of action. In scenario 2, we take the information and validate it; put it in perspective of our health status, environment, preferences, and unique genetic makeup and lifestyle; and then we consider other approaches. We need to ask ourselves the questions that our doctors should ask but don't, of ourselves. Some of these include the following:

- What is my impression about my health issue and why I'm ill?
- What do I think is causing this illness?
- What else is going on in my life that could be contributing to this illness?
- What am I willing to do to heal myself, besides implementing medical treatment?
- Am I willing to try to recover from this ailment without modern treatments from the standard medical toolbox?
- Could I, in tandem with medical treatment, use other approaches to facilitate healing?

Be curious and open to exploring options beyond modern medicine. An approach that truly resonates with your unique healing journey is out there, waiting for you, and it may not be the one your doctor recommends.

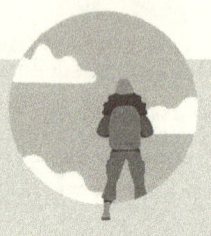

Q&A WITH ALICE: FEELING MISALIGNED WITH YOUR DOCTOR?

"I don't fully trust my doctor and sometimes feel like they're not really listening to me. Do you have any suggestions?"

It's totally natural not to click with every doctor—it happens more often than you think! We are human, and you can't expect to get along with everyone, and the same is true with your doctor. But I get where you're coming from, and it can be frustrating when you feel like your doctor isn't on the same page as you. First, try having a light but honest conversation—sometimes doctors need a little reminder to slow down and really listen. Say something like, "I'd feel more comfortable if we could discuss this a bit more." If that doesn't help, it might just be a case of mismatched personalities. In that case, don't hesitate to shop around for a doctor who better matches your style and makes you feel heard. Your health, your rules!

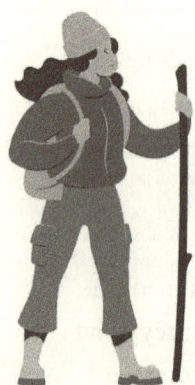

Your health, your rules!

Personalized Medicine: Tailoring Health to Your Unique Needs

In recent years, personalized medicine has gained traction as a proactive approach to health. Unlike traditional medicine, which often takes a one-size-fits-all approach, personalized medicine focuses on assessing your individual needs through advanced testing. Functional medicine providers and other specialists are at the forefront of this trend, offering services like comprehensive blood work, genetic testing, and metabolic assessments. These tests provide a detailed picture of your health, revealing potential risks and areas where you may need support long before symptoms appear.

For example, blood tests can identify nutrient deficiencies, hormone imbalances, and inflammation markers that might otherwise go unnoticed. Armed with this information, healthcare providers can make personalized recommendations, such as specific dietary changes, supplements, or lifestyle adjustments, that target your unique health profile. Genetic testing can further refine these recommendations, helping you understand your predisposition to certain conditions and how you can mitigate those risks through preventive measures.

This personalized approach isn't just for those with existing health issues—many people today are using these services to optimize their well-being and prevent potential problems down the line. In fact, the market for personalized medicine is growing rapidly, with millions of people seeking out functional medicine providers and specialized testing to tailor their health interventions. Options range from in-depth blood panels and hormone testing to DNA analysis and microbiome assessments. These tools offer valuable insights that can help you create a targeted health plan, integrating lifestyle or complementary interventions that align with your individual needs.

By leveraging modern testing and personalized recommendations, you can take control of your health in a way that's uniquely suited to you. This proactive approach not only helps mitigate risks but also empowers you to make informed decisions that support long-term wellness. Whether you're looking to optimize your health or prevent future issues, personalized medicine offers a path to more precise and effective care.

Q&A WITH ALICE: TRADITIONAL MEDICINE AND YEARS-LONG HEALTH STRUGGLES

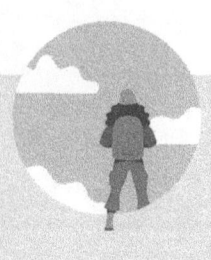

Many, many people tell they have health concerns that have gone unresolved for years, such as back pain, headaches, fatigue, anxiety, weakness, susceptibility to viruses, gut issues, etc. I often hear statements like, "I have tried everything and nothing seems to work. I guess I'll just have to live with it."

The truth is that people really *haven't* tried everything. They may have tried all the interventions prescribed by their healthcare providers, but there is no way they have tried all lifestyle changes and interventions or complementary approaches. Or they may have explored complementary practices but ignore traditional medicine alternatives.

So, my advice in this situation harkens back once again to chapter 1: Be curious. Reset your expectations, check your biases, and start over. Write down everything you've learned from whatever interventions you've tried. How did they make you feel? How did your body respond? What doesn't your body respond to, or negatively respond to? All the information gained from past experience can be used to catapult you ahead. What your body *doesn't* respond to is as important as what it *does*. Answer the questions about your health approach (chapter 11) and evaluate whether different interventions could be better aligned with your philosophy. Develop a health plan (chapter 16) that will help you try something different, or be more rigorous about implementing changes you've made in the past that were promising. Track progress, adjust, and continue to tweak your plans until you achieve your goals.

Just One Tool in Your Arsenal

I have heard many personal stories from my clients about frustrating wild goose chases they've been led on in our conventional healthcare system when trying to figure out the source of their symptoms. Referral after referral and dozens of doctor visits, tests, and pricy prescriptions later, they are left with no clear diagnosis and no suggested surefire treatment options. It's a sad story that can be rewritten.

We must be aware and prepared for the consequences of going to a modern medical provider: modern medicine leads us to one-size fits-all medical approaches. The way our healthcare system is today, doctors don't have the time to dive into our individual, unique scenario and situation. They barely have time to address our main health concern and certainly don't have time to talk about other concerns that might possibly be involved with the main concern—that would necessitate another appointment. And do they consider our unique genetic makeup, our environment, and our emotional and mental health? No way. Medical care seldom considers our personal side of health during a conventional medical treatment protocol. In general, conventional medicine is not good at managing our health from a whole-person perspective.

However, I would hope that you use good judgment and common sense when considering going to the doctor. This is not an all-or-nothing proposition. Doctors are your go-to approach for alarming, dramatic, or persistent symptoms that might indicate serious concerns, such as a malfunction of an organ or extreme illness such as repeated vomiting for long periods of time. Don't be your own doctor relying on natural remedies and miss a diagnosis of a condition that is treatable by modern medicine.

My recommendation, therefore, is that you think of traditional or conventional medicine as just ONE of the many tools you should have in your arsenal as a Health Hero. There will certainly be times when you need what modern Western medicine has to offer. But open your mind to other possibilities, as I discuss in the next chapter.

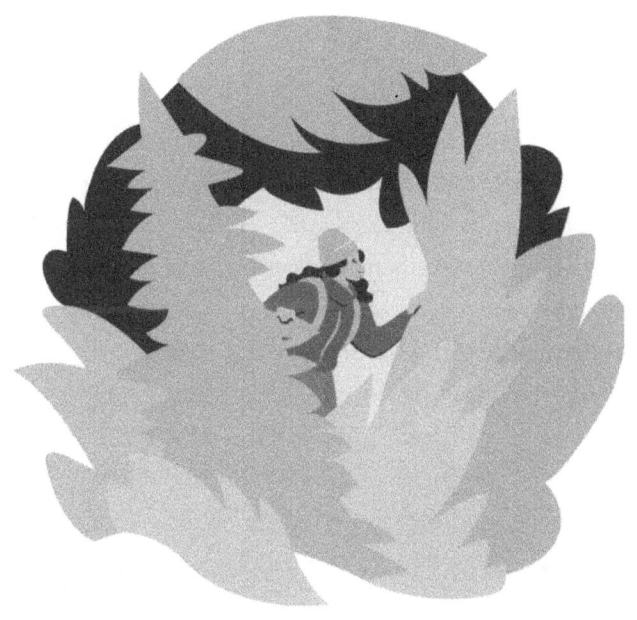

CHAPTER 15

Unlocking the Power of Complementary Healing

My own journey to go beyond the borders of conventional medicine has been driven both by what I hear from my clients and my own personal experiences. Clients with nebulous health concerns who put modern medicine on the forefront of their approach and found no relief or did not regain health led me to start questioning what was really going on. I'm referring to conditions such as fatigue, headaches, and weight gain. I experienced the same when I had my hard-to-figure health conditions, like heart palpitations and a mysterious groin pain that had no observable cause. Many times, my clients faced hopeless disappointment when they found that doctors didn't have any answers to what the cause was, nor did they have any solutions other than medication.

I've also seen individuals diagnosed with health conditions that left them without any guidance on how to reverse the condition. These folks are tagged with what traditional medicine considers to be a "forever disease," one that can only be treated with a medication, often for the rest of their lives. Being prescribed medication for a "forever disease" can feel like being handed a lifetime sentence of dependency, with no escape from potential side effects. It's a disheartening reality that no medication comes without risks, leaving the person to manage not just the disease, but also the long-term impact of the treatment itself. This path can feel limiting, as it often overlooks alternative approaches that could complement or even reduce reliance on medication. The challenge is finding ways to reclaim some control and exploring additional options that support overall well-being.

I have felt this myself when I was first diagnosed with asthma. My doctor told me, "Once an asthmatic, always an asthmatic." Is this really true? I've asked many doctors this question, and they all agree that this is the case. I've asked holistic complementary providers if they believe that I can get over my asthma symptoms, and they all emphatically say, "Yes, of course!" Who is right? I've found that both medical and complementary approaches offer valuable tools for me.

- Medical providers have prescribed me a steroid inhaler, which I use during particularly bad asthma seasons to manage symptoms effectively. They also recommended a rescue inhaler for emergencies, providing me with peace of mind.
- Complementary providers, including an acupuncturist, reflexologist, and herbalist, have suggested they could heal my asthma completely. While I haven't committed fully to testing these claims

with intense effort, I have integrated some holistic practices into my routine. For example, I use breath work techniques during asthma episodes, which are effective most of the time. I've also identified and avoided foods that trigger my asthma, helping me manage the condition more naturally.

Ultimately, a blended approach has worked best for me. It allows me to use conventional medicine when necessary, particularly in acute situations, while also exploring and benefiting from holistic methods. This balance helps me avoid medications unless absolutely needed and maintain a proactive stance in managing my health. Whether complete healing is possible through complementary practices alone remains uncertain for me, but this combined approach supports my personal health approach.

In this chapter, I walk through a number of the most popular and accessible types of complementary practices and illustrate how they can fit into your health plan even if you are still using conventional medicine as well.

New Paths to Consider

Complementary interventions encompass a spectrum of nonmainstream—sometimes referred to as unconventional—approaches, therapies, and treatments aimed at enhancing our physical, mental, and spiritual well-being, from music therapy to equine-assisted therapy. These approaches are rooted in shared principles centered on prevention, natural healing, and a mind-body-soul approach to care, offering us diverse avenues to actively participate in our health journey. Examples include approaches we are familiar with, such as acupuncture, massage therapy, hypnosis, tai chi, yoga, and mindfulness practices, to lesser-known interventions, such as biofeedback, craniosacral therapy, sound therapy, vibroacoustic therapy, moxibustion, hydrotherapy, color therapy, earthing, and art therapy. Most of these modalities are applied on their own or seamlessly integrated with modern medical interventions.

By incorporating alternative and complementary interventions into your repertoire of healthcare options, you gain the ability not only to address specific ailments but also to delve deeper into the underlying causes of health issues. Unlike traditional modern medicine, which primarily focuses on symptom management and health condition control, many complementary interventions strive to restore balance, thus fostering the conditions for healing to take place.

While the options are extensive, they can generally be categorized into various modalities, each with its own techniques and principles. Here are fourteen examples of well-known categories of alternative treatment options, listed in alphabetical order:

1. **Alternative medicine:** These medicines encompass the exploration of unconventional techniques in lieu of traditional medical methods.

2. **Ayurvedic medicine:** Also called Ayurveda, this practice seeks to bring balance back to the body's energies through consideration of the whole person, including body, mind, and spirit, in the diagnosis and treatment of disease. It takes into account an individual's physical constitution, emotional state, lifestyle, diet, and environment.

3. **Body-mind techniques:** Under professional guidance, hypnotherapy and biofeedback focus on the interplay between the mind and body to promote healing and well-being.

4. **Complementary medicine:** These include the use of additional healing and restorative approaches in tandem with conventional medicine for a more holistic approach to healing.

5. **Diet and nutrition approaches:** These approaches emphasize the role of food and nutrition in maintaining health and may include

dietary changes, nutritional supplements, and herbal remedies.

6. **Energy therapies:** Based on a concept of manipulating the body's energy fields to promote healing, they include practices such as acupuncture, Reiki, and therapeutic touch.

7. **Functional medicine:** Functional medicine is a systems biology–based approach that focuses on identifying and addressing the root causes of disease. It views the body as an interconnected system rather than separate organs and emphasizes individualized treatment plans.

8. **Herbal medicine:** Herbologists, also known as herbalists, are practitioners who specialize in the use of plants and plant extracts for medicinal purposes. They utilize their knowledge of herbs to treat a variety of health conditions, promote wellness, and maintain overall health.

9. **Integrative medicine:** Integrative medicine combines conventional Western medicine with complementary and alternative medicine practices. It seeks to treat the whole person (mind, body, and spirit) and emphasizes the therapeutic relationship between practitioner and patient.

10. **Manipulative and body-based practices:** These therapies involve physical manipulation of the body, like chiropractic care, massage therapy, and osteopathy.

11. **Mind-body practices:** These encompass techniques that focus on the connection between the mind and the body, such as meditation, yoga, tai chi, and mindfulness. Many cross over with lifestyle interventions. Those requiring a leader, teacher, or practitioner are considered complementary therapies.

12. **Naturopathy:** This natural method–driven approach harnesses the power of herbs for healing.

13. **Sensory-based therapies:** These therapies use sensory stimulation, such as aromatherapy, sound therapy, or the immersive experience of sensory deprivation to remove sound and light to promote relaxation and healing.

14. **Traditional Chinese medicine:** Traditional Chinese medicine offers a holistic approach to health that focuses on balancing the body's energies and treating the underlying causes of illness. Its various practices, from acupuncture to herbal medicine, aim to restore harmony and promote overall well-being.

There are many other complementary approaches not mentioned here that are worth exploring. Yet keep in mind that not all these therapies share the same level of scientific validation, and their impact can differ from person to person. If you choose to try complementary approaches, use a logical method to evaluate their effectiveness and safety. Be sure to use educated, credentialed, and seasoned practitioners who take into account individual health requirements, needs, and personal inclinations.

Complementary interventions can be considered a sidekick to conventional medical care, but trust is earned, not expected. I consider it as the go-to for those nebulous health conditions, such as fatigue and headaches, while allowing for medical professionals to rule out the worst-case scenario or do what they do best in emergency situations and major illnesses. But when it comes to tackling complex health problems, like seemingly irreversible diseases and mysterious symptoms, complementary approaches take the spotlight and unravel the enigma.

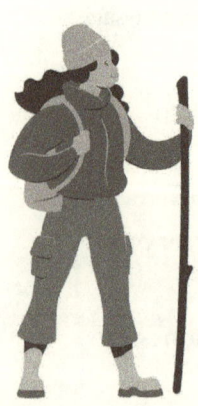

With complementary interventions, trust is earned, not expected.

Blending Traditional and Complementary Practices: A Case Study

When I began to work with clients who were not content to stop at medical treatment and decided to take more responsibility for their own healing, I saw that they needed to start by better understanding their health status. From there, I encouraged them to think with a broader vision and consider lesser-known healing options and other kinds of services that could be used to improve health.

This approach has proved fruitful over and over again. One client, Shawna, is a great example. Shawna was struggling with lower back pain, and her doctor was only able to offer muscle relaxants and pain medication, yet she desperately wanted to improve her condition without medical intervention. We then began her healing journey into the lesser-known route to healing using a wide array of healing options.

Shawna and I began our work together by having her talk about her life over the last few years. We also looked at the Health Spectrum (described in chapter 10) and discovered that she had been a Level 1: Healthy, but in the last year moved to a Level 2: Mostly Healthy, and just recently felt like she was moving into Level 3: Not as Healthy.

We discovered that her life story aligned directly with her health level movement. She was facing strong stressors at work, home, and in her personal life that began about a year ago, but which continued to escalate. Add to that, she was working most days on the computer, and sitting had always tended to aggravate her back. It became evident that her lower back was where Shawna's body was accumulating the essence of her living experience.

Taking a step back gives us more insight into why we might be feeling the way we are. Many times, we're not healthy because we're challenged beyond what we can cope with, we're overwhelmed, or we're sad. Maybe we're faced with insufferable relationships, inescapable work demands, or unhealed trauma. For me, when I am stressed, my breathing tightens—I get a mild case of asthma. My lungs are my weak spot where I accumulate all the stress and where my body holds onto it. Where is that place for you in your body? What is it that is going on in your life right now that could be showing up in susceptible aspects of your health?

I proceeded to ask Shawna what she thought her body was telling her, and her response was, "It's telling me to love it, and not push it so hard." She continued, "It's telling me that my job is the wrong job and to quit it. My job is making it sad. It's telling me that I have to say 'no' more and stop living like I don't matter. I do matter, and I have to start loving myself more. I think it's also telling me to fill my soul."

Wow . . . the body talks and if we listen to it, we can start to find new ways to heal.

If I had taken the traditional approach with Shawna that many personal trainers and lifestyle coaches would have taken, I would have put Shawna on a strength training program, assessed her office space, and had her make a few adjustments. I would have encouraged her to drink more water, eat more vegetables, and walk more. But by asking a few questions, Shawna began to come up with her own solutions, and guess what? She came up with all of those actions and more. All I had to do was ask questions that gave her the perspective and the vision for healing in the ways her body needed.

Shawna and I also went through some additional options in the realm of medical, complementary, and lifestyle approaches. She decided to table medical treatment for the time being and focus on complementary and lifestyle approaches. Her lifestyle approaches were the exact approaches I listed earlier, such as adjusting her office setting and strengthening her back and core muscles. But it also included looking for a new job, cutting out things in her life that were not aligning with her spirit, and going back to her faith in God.

Shawna also explored different complementary approaches to specifically focus on the area of her back. Shawna chose to try a massage technique called cupping. As she continued to adjust her lifestyle a little at a time, and try regularly scheduled cupping, her back began to feel incrementally better over the next six weeks. Then she moved from cupping and tried TENS therapy (transcutaneous electrical nerve stimulation)—an approach that looked promising and doable.

Over the next six weeks, Shawna went to her physical therapist and had electrode pads placed on two opposite areas of her aching back. A low electrical current was sent through the pained muscle. The procedure was not in the least painful, but afterward she felt as if her back was less tight than before. About six months after we first started working together, during our regularly scheduled call, she said, "I can't believe this, but for the first time, I forgot why I was meeting with you—my back pain is essentially gone!"

Was her relief due to the TENS therapy? Or was it the ergonomic adjustment to her workspace? Maybe it was because of her well-hydrated back muscles and lowered stress? The answer to those questions is "yes." Her relief was due to them all.

Shawna practiced a layered approach to healing, which first started by addressing the root causes of her pain. From there, each intervention Shawna tried moved the healing needle a little more back to Level 1: Healthy. Of course, it took Shawna some effort, time, resources, and patience, but her logical approach healed her faster. She also could have tried different therapies from more expensive to free, less invasive to more, but the healing likely would have been on the same trajectory. Shawna was listening to her body and paying attention. She was doing something good for herself and self-healing.

Optimizing Health: Think "And," Not "Either/Or"

How do you approach your health today? Take a moment to reflect on your current approach to health interventions. Are you more inclined toward medical, complementary, or lifestyle interventions? Is there one you rely on more than the others? How can you enhance your health strategy to create synergy among all three and move yourself into an optimal zone of health, what I call the Health Optimization Zone? (See figure 15.1.)

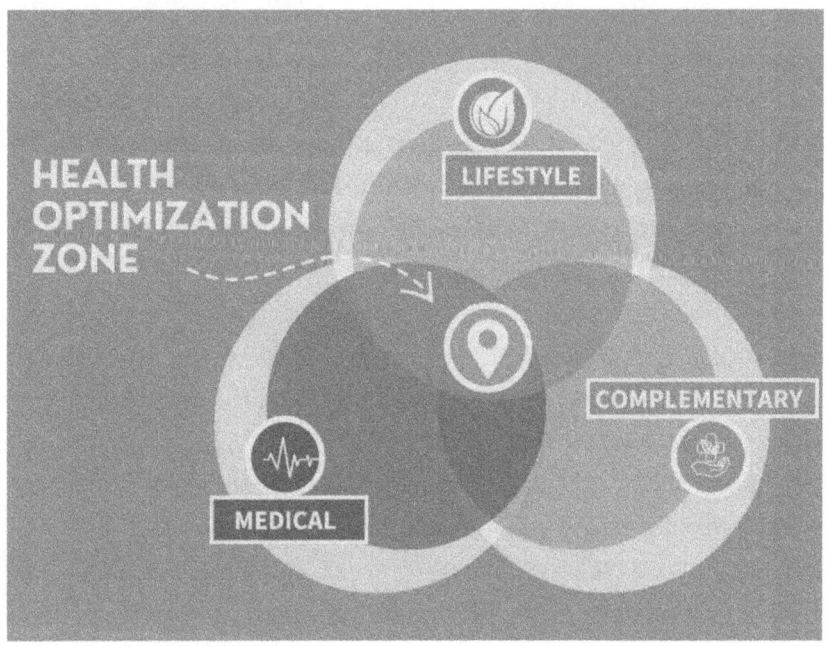

Figure 15.1: The Health Optimization Zone

Consider the formidable battle against cancer, where medical treatment often serves as the front-line assault. In this fierce encounter, chemotherapy or radiation may act as powerful weapons, targeting and dismantling cancer cells. However, these medical interventions can inadvertently wreak havoc on the body's defenses, leaving it battered and weakened in their wake.

Yet, this is precisely where complementary and lifestyle therapies can come to the rescue. Imagine acupuncture soothing the weary body, massage therapy providing relief, and a nutrient-rich diet fortifying your defenses. These allies bolster your body's recovery, helping it regain strength and vitality while minimizing the collateral damage of medical treatment. They don't just heal; they empower your body to emerge from the battle healthy. The Health Optimization Zone allows us to find the path to optimal health, and this path is always a trifecta—a convergence of medical, complementary, and lifestyle interventions. Instead of being forced to choose just one, we have the remarkable opportunity to harness the power of all three simultaneously. It's within this trifecta that health transformation accelerates and the human body becomes an incredibly resilient and adaptable force, capable of achieving remarkable feats of healing. This sweet spot is the Health Optimization Zone.

In the realm of health management, it's crucial to understand that no single path reigns supreme. Let me emphasize this again—we are all unique, and everyone has a unique set of circumstances that no one else can fully understand. We are the only ones who truly know ourselves, inside and out, and what path we should take to healing. But no matter what path we take, medical, complementary, and lifestyle interventions should be part of our healing and health management.

This central area where all three intervention types converge is the area where we can be most effective and efficient when finding ways to address our health. Here's how the optimization zone looks for each level of health.

- **Level 1: Healthy** and **Level 2: Mostly Healthy:** Medical, complementary, and lifestyle interventions all play together to keep you at your best. Use medical interventions to track your health by setting a baseline health measurement and understanding your default health. Use lifestyle and complementary interventions to keep you well and functioning optimally, and to help propel you back to Level 1: Healthy when health starts to drive to Level 2: Mostly Healthy.

- **Level 3: Not as Healthy:** You will rely more on medical interventions, but still complementary and lifestyle interventions will keep you from becoming a Level 4: Not Healthy, and lifestyle and complementary interventions might just move you back into a Level 2: Mostly Healthy. Certainly, lifestyle and complementary interventions can help you with symptom management and keep you from contracting other conditions.

- **Level 4: Not Healthy:** Your reliance on medical care is crucial, but using complementary and lifestyle interventions will keep you going, ease your pain, and possibly improve your condition, moving you into Level 3: Not as Healthy.

Although the use of the three interventions probably makes intuitive sense, many of us find ourselves grappling with limiting beliefs that suggest one intervention is superior to the rest, or that we should follow a single path, excluding the others. We may hear statements like "Complementary medicine is a waste of time and money" or "I don't trust doctors." These declarations often stem from past experiences, hearsay, or personal biases.

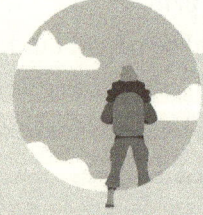

Q&A WITH ALICE: OPTIMIZING HEALTH

The concept of the Health Optimization Zone is to help people harness the power of medical, complementary, and lifestyle interventions to achieve a health goal or resolve a concern. When I introduce this concept, people will ask me, "What's the best way to get all three intervention strategies working seamlessly together and cohesively?"

My response is that, in a perfect world, all three intervention strategies would interplay and coordinate. Unfortunately, they seldom do. It's up to you to create a harmonious synergy among medical, complementary, and lifestyle interventions. Articulate your health philosophy and health approach (chapters 5 and 11) and use them to do a gut check on interventions you've decided to try. Adjust your plans and goals to resolve any conflicts. Mention the alternative approaches that you're using to your providers to keep them informed. It may sound overwhelming, but most of the time you must orchestrate what you need, when you need it. That's what it means to take control of your health destiny!

Open Minds and Limitless Possibilities

Imagine a realm of healthcare where your well-being takes center stage. A place where your active participation in your health isn't just welcomed, it's celebrated. Complementary interventions open the door to this world, offering unconventional, potentially impactful approaches to promote physical, mental, and spiritual health. From ancient practices like acupuncture and yoga to forgotten therapies like reflexology, deep breathing, tapping, and hypnotherapy, complementary approaches allow you to explore an overabundance of holistic options. These methods empower you to address not just your symptoms but the root causes of your health concerns, too.

As Health Heroes, we must resist the urge to dismiss any intervention based on preconceived notions (although some interventions *may* be found to not suit us well based on experience). Instead, keep an open mind and understand that each element of the trifecta of traditional, complementary, and alternative medicine has a role in the journey toward health and healing.

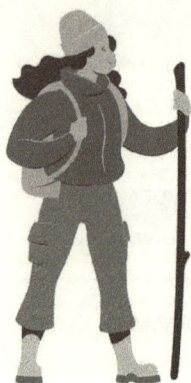

At the intersection of medical, complementary, and lifestyle interventions lives the ability to work smarter, not harder, to heal your condition.

By discarding limiting beliefs, we unlock the full potential of the synergy within the intersection of medical, complementary, and lifestyle interventions, the Health Optimization Zone, and set ourselves on a path of maximizing our best health. That is how Health Heroes handle their health: they work smarter, not harder, to heal. With this arsenal of tools from each intervention bucket at your disposal, you can navigate the complex landscape of health by harnessing the powers within each intervention.

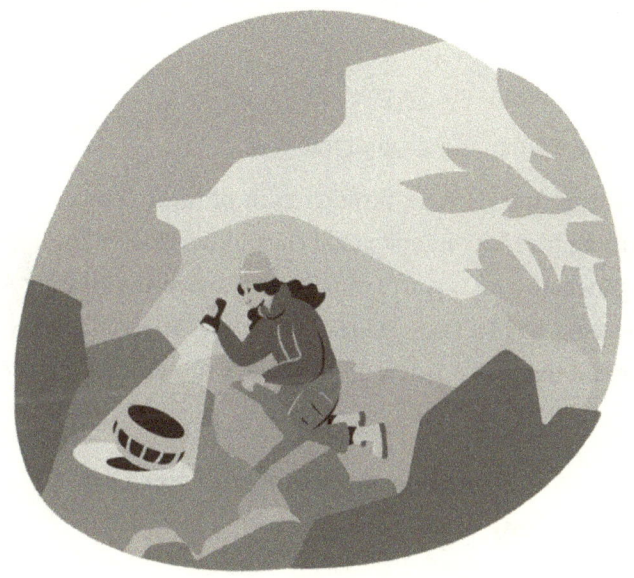

CHAPTER 16

Creating a Healing Action Plan Just for You

In chapter 5, I talk about the importance of defining your health philosophy. It's now time to keep that health philosophy in mind, as well as your health approach and goals. We're going to put them all together and make a plan to heal you from your health concern. Don't wait until later—now's the time. The sooner you start, the better your chances are for health recovery, protection, and disease reversal.

You're going to create the process to heal. Identify whatever it is that you want to work on. You will then build a Healing Action Plan created both *by* you and *for* you. A Healing Action Plan has four components:

1. Your health goal
2. Interventions, treatments, or actions you want to pursue to reach that goal
3. Expectations and targets
4. Preparation, launch, and tracking

In this chapter, I walk through each of these components (summarized in figure 16.1). I hope you'll start to develop your plan. As you go through whatever it is you're wanting to achieve, the Healing Action Plan you develop will be your guide. The process is simple, but you have to implement the plan if you want to achieve success. You can do this!

Healing Action Plan Checklist

My Health Goal
- [ ] I've identified the health issue I want to resolve or the health goal (such as fitness or nutrition) I want to achieve

Options I'm Going to Try
- [ ] I've answered the CREECS questions (commitment, risk, effectiveness, effort, cost, support)
- [ ] I've done research and checked multiple reliable sources of information to explore options from conventional medicine, complementary practices, and lifestyle interventions
- [ ] I've narrowed the list down to one to five optons to try that are consistent with my health philosophy and approach
- [ ] I've checked to ensure my biases have not unduly influenced my choices
- [ ] I'm sure I can commit to the options I've selected

Expectations and Targets
- [ ] I know what tier of intervention each option falls into and have identified expectations consistent with that tier
- [ ] I've identified SMART goals for each option (Specific, Measurable, Achievable, Relevant, Time-bound)

Preparations, Launch, Tracking
- [ ] I know what preparations I should do to increase the chances of my success
- [ ] I've identified a launch date
- [ ] I've decided how to track progress (line graphs, journal, spreadsheet, etc.)

Figure 16.1: Healing Action Plan Checklist

1. Define Your Health Goal

Decide what it is you want to resolve, or what it is you want to achieve. Typically, the goal will fall into one of two categories:

- Resolving a specific health concern (such as weight loss, joint pain, irritability, depression, headaches)
- A fitness or nutrition goal you want to reach (such as being able to walk around a block or run a 10K)

Whatever you decide, make sure the goal is something important to *you*. Check to make sure you're not being influenced in a bad way by outside parties or biases, as discussed in chapter 2.

2. Select One to Five Options to Pursue

What are the options to choose from to achieve this?

- Start by answering the CREECS questions: What are your feelings around commitment, risk, effectiveness, effort, cost, and support?
- Then do research into options and their efficacy (use the information in chapter 4 about navigating the information landscape to help you get started). Be curious! Review all the options, including medical, complementary, and lifestyle intervention ideas.
- List at least enough viable ideas to consider that align with your CREECS tolerances. No need to hold back—write down any health interventions that appeal to you and get creative! Don't throw these ideas away—you can always look back and try them later. Please consider the Core 4 (exercise, nutrition, sleep, and hydration) as part of your interventions if you haven't fully mastered any. These are foundational and will enhance the effectiveness of whatever else you try.
- Pick anywhere from one to five interventions or actions to try. Doing too much is a recipe for failure, so don't go overboard.

- Be sure to pick interventions that make sense and align with the potential cause of the condition, if possible. For example, if you choose to follow a specific diet, make sure it aligns with your current medications. Consider your unique circumstance and genetics as you peruse through the options. Lean on different personalities to find alternative approaches. Find people who have styles other than yours and ask them for their opinions.

- Double check to make sure your interventions align with your health philosophy (see chapter 5).

> ### No One Right Way
>
> Remember, there is no magic, one-way, "This is what you should do" next step. There's no right or wrong here. You may want me to tell you what to do, but what needs to happen is that you need to try an intervention—period. Try something and see how it works.

- Ask yourself one last time if you can commit to each intervention. If not, trim the list. You can always try the other options later, after you've mastered the first steps you end up taking.

One last warning: obviously, there are some interventions that are not appropriate for your health issue. I expect you are smart and logical when choosing your health interventions. Make sure they are appropriate, align well with your concern, and show efficacy in addressing your ailments or conditions. But if you're still not sure how to address your health concern, ask someone you trust who has another health decision-making style what they think, keep talking to professionals who have different perspectives on the matter, and keep looking and researching. I have no simple answer to your health ailment because you are unique and there is no one way to get you from point A to point B. There are many ways to get there; some are conventional, and some are not. Trust that you know what you need to do to improve your health. Based on what you know right now, what would be the best way to address your health issue? Try that for a while and see what happens. Track and assess your progress, which I talk about in the next section. If what you chose to try doesn't work, no worries—you can try another of the options next. You have a plan, and you're not reliant on just one approach—you have options!

3. Set Expectations and Define Targets

Managing our health is full of balancing acts. It's a balance of listening to your body and knowing what your body needs and doing what is needed to bring health and healing. It's a balance of intervening at just the right time, not too early and not too late, to pave the way for maximum healing. It's a balance of focusing attention on the most important health concerns while also continuing to support other areas of your health to maintain overall health. It's a balance of finding an intervention that comes your way at just the right time, while also not succumbing to tempting, unhelpful interventions, and being wise enough to know the difference. That's why I want you to make sure the goals you've chosen are the best aligned for your health condition.

When you're faced with a health condition, you need to focus your attention on the right interventions at the right time, or you may miss a healing opportunity, accelerate your condition, or subject yourself to wasted time and money on useless, or even detrimental, interventions. You need to know the difference between which health issues are critical to address versus which aren't. That's why I developed a way for us to see health interventions in a context of tiers of effectiveness—because not all health interventions are worth your time and money. Let's look at the four tiers (summarized in table 16.1).

- **Tier 1 interventions** are those that you must do because they're critical for your health. If your arm is dangling by a thread, you must have it sewn back on, so sewing it back on is a tier 1 intervention. If you're having a heart attack, you can't wait and try eating more salad at dinner to see if it will help—that would be ridiculous. You need to go to the emergency room and get tier 1 interventions. Tier 1 interventions are those that matter right now—you must do them. You must go see a doctor—you must take care of this health problem—or else your health will rapidly decline.

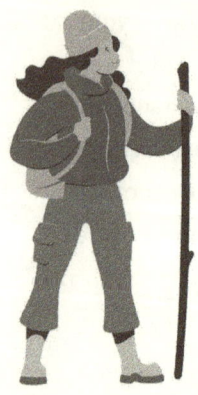

If you know what to expect, you'll save time and avoid the disappointment of false hopes.

- **Tier 2 interventions** aren't critical, but they're vital for overall health. For example, if you found out you have high blood sugar, you'll want to do something about your blood sugar soon or you'll be at risk of getting diabetes. In this example, following a mindful diet is a tier 2 intervention, as well as weight loss, if you're overweight. Those interventions make sense in addressing high blood sugar. The Core 4—nutrition, exercise, sleep, and hydration—are all tier 2 interventions because they can make or break your overall health quickly if they're not incorporated regularly into your lifestyle.

- **Tier 3 interventions** are meaningful interventions, but they're not urgent or vital. These are interventions that support our overall health; we derive enjoyment and positive effects from, such as massage, meditation, or support groups; or we find that they enhance our quality of life in some way. Implementing more than one tier 3 intervention at the same time may even collectively synergize to improve your health and help you slowly heal, although obviously it depends on the interventions you choose. Just don't expect a tier 3 intervention to reverse a disease, especially by itself. But I can't say that it's not happened; it's just not common.

- **Tier 4 interventions** are those that seldom impact our health for the better over the long haul. These interventions include the use of beauty and vanity products, such as supplements for hair regrowth or skin repair creams. Many times, tier 4 interventions are externally initiated—an ad pops up on your computer screen, or maybe a coworker urges you to try a protein supplement purported to help reduce body fat. These are perfect examples of tier 4 interventions. Being in tier 4 doesn't necessarily mean they're ineffective; they may or may not be. But regardless, they are not essential. I've seen many people try a tier 4 intervention, hoping it resolves a major health issue, when a tier 2 intervention is needed. One popular example is a bowel cleanse. These are usually a seven-to-ten-day protocol with shakes, liquids, or supplements that promise to detox and cleanse the body. The truth is that over the time frame you will eat less and so you will likely lose weight. The weight loss alone will make you feel like you're doing something good for your health. In the meanwhile, you're out hundreds of dollars. Was a bowel cleanse needed? No—it was a tier 4 intervention that made you feel good, but it didn't change your health trajectory for the better.

Out of all the interventions you're doing for your health right now, where do your health interventions fall within the tiers? Are you susceptible to trying tier 4 interventions when they cross your path? If so, do you really need them or think they're worthwhile? Take time to consider tier 4 interventions in light of usefulness and cost.

TIERS OF INTERVENTIONS	DESCRIPTION	EXAMPLES
Tier 1	Critical interventions needed immediately to address serious health issues	Emergency surgery, immediate medical care
Tier 2	Vital interventions that are important for overall health but not immediately critical	Managing high blood pressure, high blood sugar, or other health conditions that have potential lifelong ramifications; Core 4
Tier 3	Meaningful interventions that support overall health and well-being but are not urgent or vital	Massage, meditation, support groups, activities that enhance quality of life
Tier 4	Interventions that seldom impact long-term health, often externally initiated, and not essential	Beauty regimens, vanity supplements, nonessential programs, such as those found with weight loss or related to detox or cleansing

Table 16.1: Tiers of Intervention

Aligning Intervention Types to Meet Your Needs

When considering health interventions, it's crucial to understand how medical, complementary, and lifestyle approaches fit into the four tiers. Each type of intervention has its place, depending on the severity and nature of your health condition.

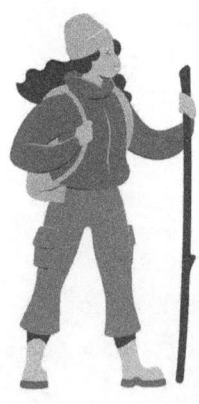

Tier 1 is essential. Tiers 2 and 3 hold opportunities, and tier 4 is purely optional.

- **Medical interventions:** Typically, medical interventions are predominantly tier 1 and tier 2. These include critical, lifesaving treatments and necessary medical procedures. For example, if you're experiencing a heart attack, immediate medical attention and intervention are crucial (tier 1). Managing chronic conditions like diabetes or rheumatoid arthritis requires regular medical checkups, medications, and specific treatments (tier 2). However, some medical interventions, like cosmetic surgeries or nonessential procedures (e.g., Botox), are in tier 4 and often are pursued for vanity rather than health necessity.

- **Complementary interventions:** Complementary interventions, such as acupuncture, chiropractic care, and herbal supplements, often fall into tier 2 and tier 3. They can play a vital role in supporting overall health and complementing primary medical treatments. For instance, acupuncture might be used alongside traditional pain management techniques to enhance relief and promote healing (tier 2). Complementary interventions are also valuable for overall well-being, such as regular massages for stress reduction (tier 3). They provide meaningful support without being critical or urgent.

- **Lifestyle interventions:** Lifestyle interventions are foundational to maintaining and improving health, often fitting into tier 2 and tier 3. These include regular exercise, balanced nutrition, adequate sleep, and proper hydration. They are essential for preventing and managing many health conditions (tier 2) and contribute significantly to overall wellness. Activities like meditation, mindfulness, and social support groups enhance quality of life and mental health (tier 3). While lifestyle interventions might not provide immediate results, their cumulative effect is profound and vital for long-term health.

- **Matching interventions to health conditions:** The severity and urgency of your health condition should guide your choice of interventions. For acute, life-threatening conditions, immediate medical interventions (tier 1) are necessary. For chronic but manageable conditions, a combination of medical and complementary interventions (tier 2) is often required to stabilize and improve health. For maintaining general well-being and enhancing quality of life, lifestyle and complementary interventions (tier 3) are highly effective. It's essential to critically evaluate the potential benefits and costs of tier 4 interventions, ensuring they align with your health goals and do not distract from more impactful treatments.

By understanding the tiers and types of interventions, you can make informed decisions that match the urgency and nature of your health needs, boosting your chances of effective healing and long-term wellness. Without this alignment, healing may remain out of reach if you rely on interventions that don't truly address your needs.

Setting Goals

Make SMART health goals for each intervention you've chosen, shaped by realistic expectations. SMART goals are a powerful tool for achieving your health objectives. They remind you to set goals that are **specific, measurable, achievable, relevant,** and **time-bound.** By clearly defining what you want to accomplish, tracking your progress, ensuring your goals are realistic, focusing on what matters most, and setting a deadline, you're more likely to stay on track and succeed in your health journey.

4. Prepare, Act, and Track

Determine what it is that you need to do to prepare. For example, make a doctor's appointment, get a gym membership or personal trainer, buy a journal, throw away processed foods and purchase healthy foods, get a support buddy, or find a therapist.

Then pick a launch date—the time when you actually employ your intervention and give it time to show its helpfulness in addressing your health concerns.

Be sure to also pick an end date, at least six weeks out. This will give you some idea of whether the intervention is helping. You can always continue the intervention after the six weeks, even if it's not showing results right away—you can decide if you want to continue trying that intervention or if you're ready to try an alternative one instead.

Once you've started, you need to track your progress. That may not sound thrilling, but it's actually a secret weapon for success. Think of it like keeping score in a game—you wouldn't want to play without knowing if you're winning, right? By jotting down your results, you're not just measuring the effectiveness of your health interventions, you're celebrating the small victories along the way. It's like giving yourself a high five every time you see improvement. Plus, tracking helps you spot any bumps in the road early on, so you can course-correct before things get off track. And let's be honest, there's nothing quite as satisfying as seeing your hard work pay off in real time. The next section describes a number of tools you can use to track progress and visualize your progress.

Why is tracking important? Many times, people begin a health intervention and lose enthusiasm and momentum somewhere around week three in a six-week trial because they're not seeing progress. Progress fuels the passion to continue. But not every intervention will produce outwardly visible progress. Sometimes our health interventions are working under the surface and haven't tipped the scale to be seen outwardly just yet.

For example, it's not uncommon for a client who starts on a strength-training and nutrition-focused weight loss effort to get discouraged halfway though. Even though they look better and feel better, they get discouraged because the scale hasn't revealed progress. Body fat analysis shows that their body fat has indeed shifted to less fat and more muscle, but they can't see the progress, so they begin to get discouraged.

So, what do you do when this happens? Decide to stick with it. Keep going and stay fully committed to the six weeks or whatever time frame you've given your intervention to take effect.

If you aren't seeing quick progress, remember that true healing often takes time and requires patience and perseverance. Instant results are rare, and just because you don't see immediate improvement doesn't mean healing isn't happening. Focus on small, incremental changes that you can see when you track your progress, and recognize that these minor victories are stepping stones to larger success.

While you are trying a health intervention, remember that your goal is not perfection, it's progress. It's not the how you get there that matters, but that you get there, and the progress will look different for everyone.

> ### Celebrate!
>
> Well, that's it! You've now worked through all four components of a Healing Action Plan. Celebrate having a plan . . . then celebrate the milestones you pass as you implement and track your progress.

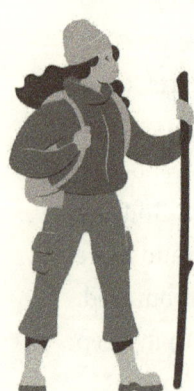

Progress fuels passion to continue.

How to Track Your Progress

Tracking will help you gauge progress and know if the intervention is working.[1] But just what should you track? The answer is, it depends on the intervention you choose, and the health concern you're working on. It also depends on how much effort you're willing to put into tracking. I give you several options to choose from. Pick the one that you know you will commit to for your entire six-week journey to healing.

What should you track? If you want to lose weight, track your weight over time. Track pain or strength if you're hoping to heal from an injury. If you implement the Core 4's exercise goal, then track steps or time spent exercising. Invest in a wearable device, like a smartwatch, which can now record your heart rate, oxygen saturation, and even sleep patterns. Or you can take photos as you go along, too. Just be sure to track something that measures your progress.

Measuring Biometrics

For some health goals, tracking biometric data like weight, body fat, waist circumference, blood pressure, blood values like blood glucose and cholesterol, body temperature, and heart rate and rhythm are crucial to see what is happening physiologically with your intervention. Like I mention before, biofeedback devices like HeartMath heart rhythm monitors can give you an understanding of your stress levels from a biometric perspective, too. There are now apps like Daylio that can help you track your mood and activities to identify emotional patterns, too. Many apps have a free version, too.

Line Chart

Line charts are one of my favorite health navigation tools because they are a simple and efficient tool that helps us quantify our concerns and allows us to visualize how we feel over time (see figure 16.2). Line charts can detect trends, correlations, and other events that might impact how we feel and assist us to better notice and understand ourselves.

Weekly Progress Line Graph

The health concern I want to improve:
....
....

The intervention I'm using:
....

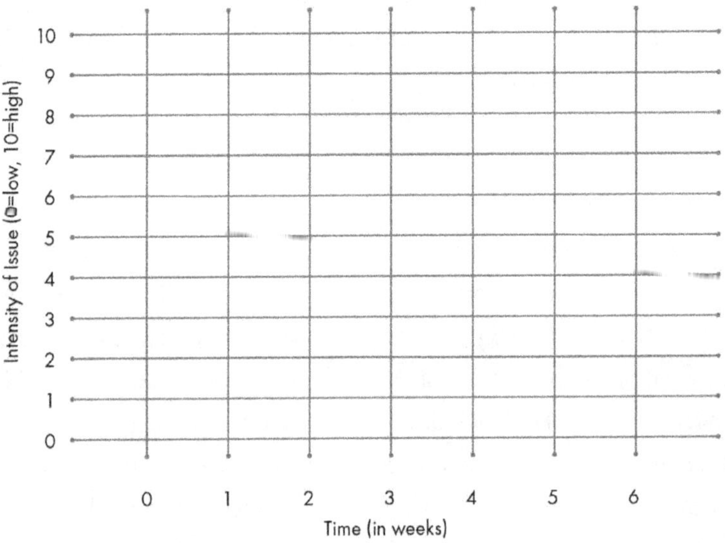

[Line graph with Y-axis labeled "Intensity of Issue (0=low, 10=high)" ranging from 0 to 10, and X-axis labeled "Time (in weeks)" ranging from 0 to 6]

Figure 16.2: Format for Tracking Progress on a Line Graph

Charting our food and mood is a great example. Because food has such a powerful influence on our health and mood, a line chart can be a great way to visualize if and how our eating impacts how we feel physically and emotionally. Figure 16.3 is an example of how you can track how you feel with what you eat during the day.

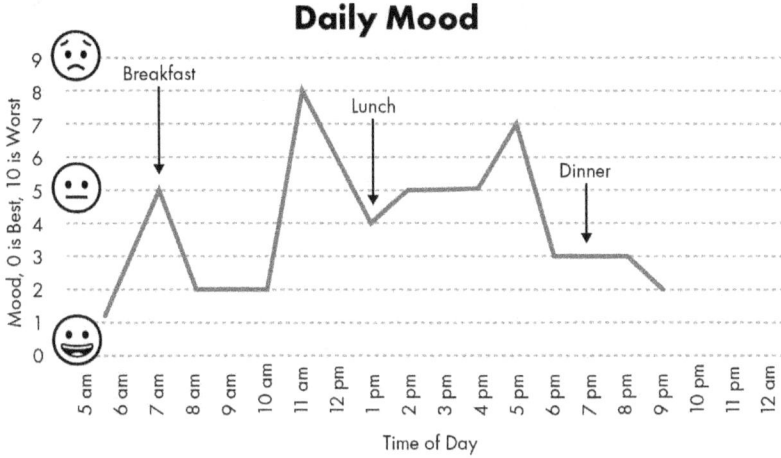

Figure 16.3: Line Graph Showing Daily Mood Swings

Depending on your needs, you can choose to graph daily, monthly, or even annually to get an idea of how your mood changes throughout a short or long time period. Line charts can be used to track mood or symptom strength with other possible correlating factors, too. For example, line charts would be an easy way to track mood and seasons throughout the year, as seen in figure 16.4. What is revealed in the chart can enlighten us to supplement mood-enhancing activities or interventions to offset times when spirits are lower, such as increasing vitamin D or taking mini-vacations. Of course, not everything needs to be charted, only issues or concerns that we are curious about or concerned about the most. Suggestions include tracking correlations between physical activity and sleep, food and energy, or drinking caffeine and irritability. Line charts are a great way to learn more about yourself and how you continue to change over a lifetime, too. There are endless uses for the simple line chart to bring self-awareness to facilitate self-discovery and healing.

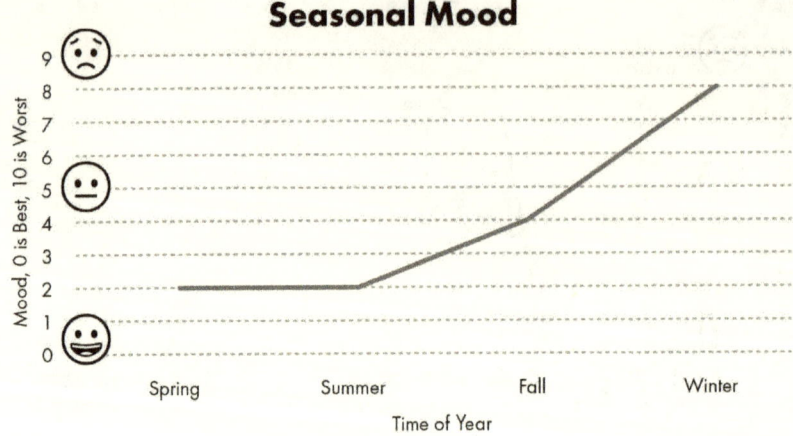

Figure 16.4: Line Graph Tracking Seasonal Mood Swings

Health Data Journaling

If you choose to be more old-school and less techy with your tracking, start to keep a journal where you track your health information. Write down your symptoms or changes daily, including what you ate, how you slept, and your stress or pain levels. I've included a Health Journal page that you can copy and use, or find one online if you'd like to be reminded to record the basics using a no-thinking-needed template (see figure 16.5).

Daily Health Journal

My health mantra: _____

Date: _____ How am I doing today? 😊 😐 ☹️

Focus: _____ How am I doing today compared with yesterday? (Worse, same, better, new symptoms . . .) Explain:

Lifestyle intervention(s) today: _____

Complementary intervention(s) today: _____ Activity yesterday vs today? (More active, no exercise yesterday vs exercise today . . .)

Medical intervention(s) today: _____ Type of activity: _____

Symptoms I'm Tracking

Symptom:	Same/Better/Worse than yesterday:
●	Same/Better/Worse
●	Same/Better/Worse
●	Same/Better/Worse
●	Same/Better/Worse

Energy 😊 😐 ☹️
Sleep last night 😊 😐 ☹️
Mood 😊 😐 ☹️
Pain 😊 😐 ☹️
Appetite 😊 😐 ☹️
Stress 😊 😐 ☹️
Sick 😊 😐 ☹️
Activity yesterday Low/Medium/High
Activity today Low/Medium/High
How hydrated am I? 💧 💧 💧

Anything Else?
_____
_____
_____
_____
_____

Medicines and Supplements

What/Amount:	
●	AM/Midday/PM
●	AM/Midday/PM
●	AM/Midday/PM
●	AM/Midday/PM
●	AM/Midday/PM

Today was **Same/Better/Worse** than yesterday

Figure 16.5: Daily Health Journal Format

Journaling is one of the best ways to capture multiple facets of your healing journey, including feelings. I made a simple Daily Health Journal, too, that you can use right now to start to see your health transformation begin in real time.

Spreadsheets

Spreadsheets are also a great way to track multiple variables simultaneously over time. Make a date column with every day listed, then make columns for weight, mood, pain, sleep—whatever it is you want to track. Type in your results at the end of each day and create a graph or chart weekly to bring it to life. Check out the example for Meg in table 16.2.

DATE	WEIGHT	MOOD (1-10)	PAIN (1-10)	SLEEP QUANTITY, (HOURS)
08/24/24	150	6	3	7
08/30/24	149.5	7	3	7.5
09/5/24	148.8	7	2	8
09/10/24	148.5	8	1	9
09/14/24	148	7	2	7.5
09/20/24	147.7	8	2	8

Table 16.2: Example of a Spreadsheet for Meg

In this example, Meg decided to take a more organized approach to her health by using a spreadsheet to track the impact of her interventions. She set up simple columns for weight, mood, pain levels, and sleep, and instead of logging every day, she recorded her data a few times a week. This allowed her to see how her efforts were paying off without feeling overwhelmed by daily tracking.

By using the spreadsheet, Meg noticed patterns she hadn't seen before—like how her mood improved when she got more sleep or how her pain levels dropped after making certain dietary changes. The visual progress on her spreadsheet helped her stay motivated and keep with her interventions based on real data. Over time, Meg found that this method gave her a clearer understanding of what worked for her, helping her make better health decisions and stay on track toward her goals. You can expand this table with more days and any additional health factors you want to monitor, too.

Taking a broader view of your health by tracking progress over time is incredibly valuable. You don't need to track every single day—just enough to notice patterns and see how your efforts are paying off. By focusing on the bigger picture, you can gain meaningful insights into what's working and make adjustments as needed. Remember, it's about progress, not perfection, so track at a pace that feels sustainable and encouraging. This way, you'll stay motivated and see the positive changes unfold over time.

> ### You Can't Measure What You Don't Track
>
> As you can see, there are many ways to track your progress, but the key is to just track something. How do you know if your health interventions are working? Subjective day-to-day feelings can be misleading, and in our busy lives, we forget what we don't track. This is your chance to learn more about how your body responds to health interventions so that you can use that knowledge to your advantage. For example, say hypnosis didn't work, but a Theta Pod did. You can start to get a sense for where the health concern is originating from and what your body can use to recover. This transformation begins with data—track, track, track.

Remember: Believe That You Can Heal

Before closing out this chapter, let me pause for just a second. I want to remind you of something that is more important than implementing all the components of your Healing Action Plan. It is the need to have a mindset shift—the belief that you can be healthy again—that you can lose weight, recover from the illness, help your family member get better, and return to a healthy life. Doubt may start creeping in, making you question if it can be done. That is a normal thought because we can't see the future, so it's hard to put faith in something we can't see. But you are no longer ordinary; you are a Health Hero, equipped to take on the healing challenge armed with every tool you need!

So, when fear and doubt creep in, remember that they are a safety mechanism that our brains use to keep us safe—they are normal responses. When this happens, stop and breathe and tell yourself that this is a situation that requires resetting the mind to neutral, and then begin to apply logic and reason to navigate the next steps.

Remember, your thoughts will ultimately shape your results because your thoughts are the driving force behind your feelings, which influence your actions, and your actions produce your results. Do you see how we have the power to heal with our minds? The Core 4 are fundamental for our well-being, and managing our stress, environment, and financial life are all important for optimizing and maximizing our overall health. But when it comes to healing from an illness, belief reigns supreme. Remember, the goal is to have a mindset that you will heal.

I've witnessed how a mindset shifts to believing you can heal someone over and over again, in spite of what doctors said. For example, a client of mine had problems with low bowel motility. Her doctor and dietitian told her that she couldn't eat foods high in fiber, like fresh fruits and vegetables, only cooked veggies, for the rest of her life. Her dissatisfaction with that possibility led her to create a Healing Action Plan that included herbs, reflexology, gentle strategic exercise, and massage, and today she is eating normal foods again without any gut issues. She gave her body the chance to heal, believed it could heal, and so she pursued healing.

Another client suffered with a chronic shoulder injury after trying physical therapy with no relief. His doctor told him that surgery was inevitable if he wanted to relieve his pain. We talked about his options, and he decided to try to heal it once again, one last time, before committing to surgery. He told himself he could heal, and so, after embarking on a six-month healing journey with a Healing Action Plan of robust physical therapy exercises with me, strategic rest, and massage, he recovered completely in five months.

There are so many stories I can share of people who put together a plan to accomplish recovery and fully recovered, or they achieved their goals. I believe the actions they chose were necessary, but believing they could heal was the secret. These clients, and so many more, have now committed to a life practice of being a Health Hero.

Your Health, Your Way

In a world of nearly eight billion souls, there is only one you—unique, exceptional, and utterly irreplaceable. Your health journey is also unique. You get to choose what you want to do with it, no one else. And you get to believe that you can heal—no one can take that away from you. I don't know about you, but I'd rather die believing I can heal than die feeling like I couldn't ever recover.

I give you permission to be fearless in your approach to healing. Give it your all and move from confusion to action using all of the knowledge that you've gained in this book. Becoming more self-aware; finding quality health information; knowing your health philosophy; picking interventions from the unlimited sources in lifestyle, complementary, and medical interventions; and tracking your results—all of these move you from confusion to decisiveness. You are in control of your health. Own it, and make healing happen.

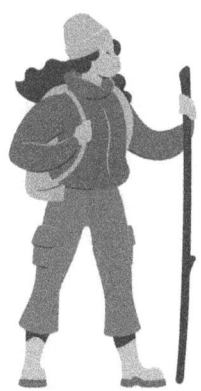

Changes in how you nurture your health is evidence that you've become a true Health Hero.

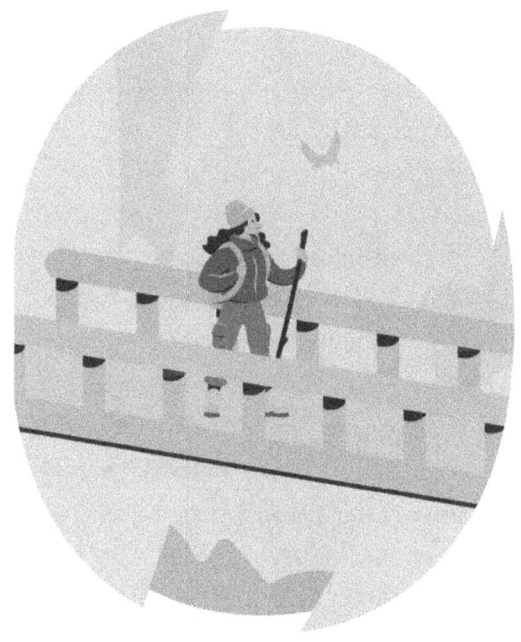

CONCLUSION

Envisioning the Journey to a HEALTHIER You

As you come to the close of this book, I want to celebrate with you. This journey I'm hoping you'll embark on is about much more than tackling a specific health condition or reaching a fitness goal—it is about recognizing that you are the hero of your own health. Your story will have a beginning, middle, and triumphant end, and the road map in this book was designed to guide you through each phase. Let's zoom out and see what I call the HEALTHIER Journey. The HEALTHIER

Journey is an acronym for the road map you can follow to improved health and confidence that you can make better health decisions.

H is for "Help Needed." This is the moment of realization—a powerful acknowledgment that you need help getting healthier. You show the courage to face where you are, which is the first step in any hero's journey. Whether you're battling a disease like cancer or vague symptoms like anxiety, sleep issues, or gut issues, this will always be your starting point. Your awareness is your first victory.

E stands for "Emotion Check." You will take a deep breath here. Before charging into action, give yourself permission to process your emotions. This is where many people falter, letting fear, frustration, or biases cloud their judgment. But not you. You will have the tools to work through these emotions and, even more importantly, establish your health philosophy, focusing on becoming confident about your ability to heal. This emotional grounding will fuel your journey from here forward.

With your emotions in check, it is time for **A**, "Acquire Information." Like any great hero, you want to become equipped with the knowledge of where you stand. But to move forward, you need more information. You will gather information about potential solutions, interventions, and ideas to help address your health. You will consider working on the Core 4 to establish a strong foundation.

Then will come **L**, "Learn More." As I've discussed many times, curiosity will be your superpower. You won't just accept the first piece of information you come across—you will dig deeper, ask questions, and continue to explore. What else could be contributing to your health issue? What are you missing? By staying curious, you can unlock new pathways for healing.

At **T**, it's time to "Think It Through." With all your new knowledge in hand, you can bring objectivity to the table using decision-making tools that strip away emotional bias. You will no longer be swayed by what's easiest or most appealing. Instead, you will make a clear, well-thought-out decision about your next steps.

Then will come the exciting part—**H**, "Head Out." You develop a Healing Action Plan, including your goals. It provides the marching orders you need to move forward and heal. You will be armed with the best personalized interventions, lifestyle changes, and tools to confidently begin your healing journey.

As you move along in your plan, **I** is for "Inspect Progress." This is where you will track your progress. Because healing isn't often instantaneous, progress has to be measured. You track your results, look at your goals, and watch and listen to your body respond to the interventions.

At **E**, you will "Evaluate Improvement." Once the time frame you selected for your plan is completed, assess your progress. Did your approach work? Are you getting better? If so, you can now continue with your plan. If not, don't worry—you still have other strategies waiting. Revisit the information you gathered and begin the next phase of your healing journey.

Finally, you will reach **R**, "Restored Health." This is the culmination of your hard work, perseverance, and dedication. You will have conquered your health challenge, and more than that, you've grown. Your character has been strengthened, and you've earned the title of Health Hero. You will look back on your journey with pride—you've gained a new perspective, resilience, and strength, not just physically but mentally and emotionally.

The HEALTHIER Journey is your forever road map to becoming healthier faster. Each step represents a key phase in your hero's journey, and each victory brings you closer to restored health and a life of well-being. With the knowledge, mindset, and tools you've gained from this book, you're now equipped to face any health challenge with confidence and clarity.

But this journey isn't just for you. The road map you've now mastered can become a powerful tool to help guide the people you love through their own health challenges. Whether it's a spouse, a parent, a child, or a friend who's struggling with their health, you now have the ability to support them as a guide or advocate. You can share the wisdom, steps, and strategies from this book, helping them identify where they are, navigate through emotions, and make informed decisions. Your knowledge is now a beacon for others who may not yet see their way through. By offering them this road map, you're empowering them to take charge of their health journey, just as you've done with yours.

This is just the beginning. You are now the Health Hero of your own health story and a potential guide for others. Keep moving forward—there is always more to discover, more ways to grow, and more opportunities to master yourself.

Remember, no one can do this for you like you can. It's time to take hold of your health destiny. When we adopt health humility, we admit that we don't have all the answers. But that's okay—because the door to healing opens when we're willing to ask new questions and explore new solutions. As you'll learn, it's not just about treatments or therapies—it's about becoming self-aware, questioning old habits, and embracing the fact that healing is possible.

I sincerely believe this book can guide you through your health journey. The U.S. healthcare system and culture may be stacked against you, but by arming yourself with the HEALTHIER Journey, you can break free from their pull and old patterns and forge your unique path to healing. You are not just a one-size, one-solution patient or health consumer—you are a wise and courageous Health Hero! Go forth and be well!

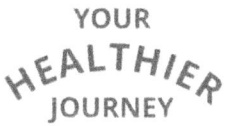

Acknowledgments

To Erin Tarectecan, thank you for your never-ending support, valuable feedback, your intertwined spirit with mine, and your ability to enter into the spirit of this project. I am beyond grateful; this book could not have been completed without you at the helm alongside me.

This book was challenging to conceive, let alone complete. The unwavering support and encouragement of my family, particularly my husband, Keith, and my children, were the fuel that propelled this project to the finish line and into the world. Thank you for being my rock! I want to express my heartfelt gratitude to Phil Lashley for his invaluable contribution in transforming the health navigation process into a meaningful and beautiful journey.

My Health Navigator Group Think Tank, specifically, Sabryna Liddle—thank you for your encouragement and support. I overcame the saboteurs, and here it is. Take that!

Notes

Introduction

1. Centers for Disease Control and Prevention. (2024, May 15). *Living with a chronic condition*. U.S. Department of Health and Human Services. https://www.cdc.gov/chronic-disease/living-with/index.html

Part I

1. AAPA. *U.S. adults spend eight hours monthly coordinating healthcare, find system "overwhelming."* (2023, May 17). https://www.aapa.org/news-central/2023/05/u-s-adults-spend-eight-hours-monthly-coordinating-healthcare-find-system-overwhelming/
2. New University of Warwick. (2022, March 31). *Subsidy would improve fruit and veg intake by as much as 15%, new research shows*. [Press release]. https://warwick.ac.uk/fac/soc/economics/research/centres/cage/news/31-03-22-subsidy_would_improve_fruit_and_veg_intake_by_as_much_as_15_new_research_shows/

Chapter 1

1. MacKrill, K., Witthöft, M., Wessely, S., & Petrie, K. J. (2023). Health scares: Tracing their nature, growth and spread. *Clinical Psychology in Europe*, 5(4). https://doi.org/10.32872/cpe.12209
2. Loney, S. (2018, December 21). *In denial: Why do we often ignore medical symptoms, when we know better?* Chatelaine. https://chatelaine.com/health/denial-ignoring-symptoms/
3. Scarantino, A. (2024). *The Routledge handbook of emotional theory*. Routledge. https://doi.org/10.4324/9781315559940
4. Eysenbach, G., & Köhler, C. (2002). How do consumers search for and appraise health information on the world wide web? Qualitative study using focus groups, usability tests, and in-depth interviews. *BMJ (Clinical research ed.)*, 324(7337), 573–577. https://doi.org/10.1136/bmj.324.7337.573

5. Bradley, E., & Taylor, L. (2015). *The American health care paradox: Why spending more is getting us less*. Public Affairs.
6. Dweck, C. S. (2006). *Mindset: The new psychology of success*. Random House.

Chapter 2

1. I've researched many places to uncover the biases against our health but always come back to these three, which are complete with resources to all the rest: Kahneman, D. (2011). *Thinking, fast and slow*. Farrar, Straus and Giroux; Kahneman, D., Sibony, O., & Sunstein, C. R. (2021). *Noise: A flaw in human judgment*. Little, Brown Spark; Pinker, S. (2021). *Rationality: What it is, why it seems scarce, why it matters*. Viking.
2. Sali, V., & Anitha, B. (2023). Impact of visual elements of packing on consumer buying behaviour of FMCG products. *UGC Care Group 1 Journal*, *51*(2), 166-172. https://www.researchgate.net/publication/375692533_IMPACT_OF_VISUAL_ELEMENTS_OF_PACKAGING_ON_CONSUMER_BUYING_BEHAVIOUR_OF_FMCG_PRODUCTS

Chapter 3

1. Serbin, L., Hubert, M., Hastings, P., Stack, D., & Schwartzman, A. (2014). The influence of parenting on early childhood health and health care utilization. *Journal of Pediatric Psychology*, *39*(10), 1161–1174. doi.org/10.1093/jpepsy/jsu050
2. Dluhos-Sebesto, C., Jethwa, T. E., Bertasi, T. G. O., Bertasi, R. A. O., Mruoka NIshi, L. Y., Pantin, S. A. L., Argenio, S. L., Shashsamand, A., Omolulu, A., & Pujalte, G. G. A., (2021). Women's health information survey: Common health concerns and trusted sources of health information among different populations of female patients. *Women's Health Reports*, *2*(1). https://doi.org/10.1089/whr.2020.0118
3. Macias, W. (2023). Women as American Family's health advocate, guide, or guardian: A health communication practitioner's perspective. *Frontiers in Communication*, *8*, 1273514. https://doi.org/10.3389/fcomm.2023.1273514
4. Ness, D. (2014, May 9). *What do mothers need? Tools to make the best health care choices*. National Partnership for Women & Families. https://nationalpartnership.org/what-do-mothers-need-tools-to-make-the-best-health-care-choices/
5. Mahmood, L., Flores-Barrantes, P., Moreno, L. A., Manios, Y., & Gonzalez-Gil, E. M. (2021). The influence of parental dietary behaviors and practices on children's eating habits. *Nutrients*, *13*(4). https://doi.org/10.3390/nu13041138
6. Williamson, L. (2024, April 17). *Families often have chief medical officers, and they're almost always women*. American Heart Association. https://www.heart.org/en/

news/2024/04/17/families-often-have-chief-medical-officers-and-theyre-almost-always-women

Chapter 4

1. Grind, K., Schechner, S., McMillan, R., & West, J. (2019, November 15). How Google interferes with its search algorithms and changes your results. *The Wall Street Journal.* https://www.wsj.com/articles/how-google-interferes-with-its-search-algorithms-and-changes-your-results-11573823753
2. American Diabetes Association Professional Practice Committee. (2024). *Introduction and Methodology: Standards of Care in Diabetes—2024.* American Diabetes Association. https://doi.org/10.2337/dc24-SINT
3. Freling, T., Yang, Z., Saini, R., Itani, O., & Abualsamh, R. (2020). When poignant stories outweigh cold hard facts: A meta-analysis of the anecdotal bias. *Organizational Behavior and Human Decision Processes, 160,* 51–67. https://doi.org/10.1016/j.obhdp.2020.01.006.

Chapter 6

1. Flynn, K., & Smith, M. (2007). Personality and health care decision-making style. *The Journals of Gerontology: Series B, 62*(5), 261–267. https://doi.org/10.1093/geronb/62.5.P261
2. Decision Aids have been helpful in many areas, including retail. There is much to learn from business marketing. This article was one of many I used to create the Four Styles of Decision-Making found in this book: Verdi, P., Kalro, A., & Sharma, D. (2019). Online decision aids: The role of decision-making styles and decision-making stages. *International Journal of Retail and Distribution Management.* Bradford, *48*(6), 555–574. https:// doi.org/10.1108/IJRDM-02-2019-0068

Chapter 7

1. I have carefully evaluated numerous decision-making tools and rigorously tested them with many of my students and clients. Each tool has its own unique strengths and weaknesses, and I can confidently say that I put them all through a comprehensive SWOT analysis! While these tools were originally designed for complex business projects, I saw the potential to adapt some of them to health management, creating a more strategic approach to making informed health decisions.

Chapter 8

1. This article is a short overview of positive psychology with references: National Institutes of Health. (2015, August). *Positive emotions and your health*. NIH News in Health. https://newsinhealth.nih.gov/2015/08/positive-emotions-your-health
2. There are many studies on the placebo and nocebo effects. If you're interested in learning more, I suggest you read this book and pay particular attention to the references: Rankin, L. (2013). *Mind over medicine: Scientific proof that you can heal yourself.* Hay House.
3. There is a wealth of research demonstrating that we can significantly enhance our performance by strategically shifting our mindset. This book draws heavily on Intentional Change Theory, emphasizing that we have the ability to coach ourselves toward meaningful growth. The following are some of the key studies and insights that have convinced me this concept is crucial—so much so that I've dedicated nearly an entire chapter to it: Baum, A., Revenson, T. A., & Singer, J. E. (Eds.). (2012). *Handbook of health psychology* (2nd ed.). Psychology Press; Boyatzis, R.E. (2019). *Coaching with intentional change theory*. In English, S., Sabatine, J. M., & Brownell, P. (Eds.), *Professional coaching: Principles and practice* (pp. 221–230). Springer Publishing Company; Reed, A., Mikels, J., & Löckenhoff, C. (2012). Choosing with confidence: Self-Efficacy and preferences for choice. *Judgement and Decision Making*, 7(2), 173–180.
4. Dominguez, L., Veronese, N., & Barbagallo, M. (2024). The link between spirituality and longevity. *Aging Clinical and Experimental Research*, (36)32. https://doi.org/10.1007/s40520-023-02684-5
5. Munnangi, S., Sundjaja, J. H., Singh, K., Dua, A., & Angus, L. D. *Placebo Effect*. (2023, November 13). StatPearls [Internet]. https://www.ncbi.nlm.nih.gov/books/NBK513296/
6. Kiecolt-Glaser, J., McGuire, L., Robles, T., & Glaser, R. (2002). Psychoneuroimmunology: Psychological influences on immune function and health. *Journal of Consulting and Clinical Psychology*, 70(3), 537–547. https://doi.org/10.1037/0022-006X.70.3.537

Chapter 9

1. Ferrer, R., Klein, W., Lerner, J., Reyna, V., & Keltner, D. (2016). Emotions and health decision-making. In C. Roberto & I. Kawachi (Eds.), *Behavioral Economics and Public Health* (pp. 101–132); Harvard University Press. Ghosh, O., & Raj, M. S. S. (2024). The vital role of emotions in health decision-making. In K. J. Reddy (Ed.), Behavioral economics and neuroeconomics of health and healthcare (pp. 299-332). IGI Global. https://doi.org/10.2337/dc24-SINT
2. Gee, C. J. (2010). How does sport psychology actually improve athletic performance? A framework to facilitate athletes' and coaches' understanding. *Behavior Modification*, 34(5), 386–402.

Chapter 10

1. I offer a couple of interesting reads on this topic: Mayer, E. (2016). *The mind-gut connection.* (pp. 8-25). HarperCollins Publishers. Dietert, R. R. (2016). *The human superorganism: How the microbiome is revolutionizing the pursuit of a healthy life.* Dutton.

Chapter 11

1. Montero, A., Sparks, G., Presiado, M., Hamel, L. (2024, May). KFF Health Tracking Poll May 2024: The Public's Use and Views of GLP-1 Drugs. *KFF.* Kaiser Family Foundation. https://www.kff.org/health-costs/poll-finding/kff-health-tracking-poll-may-2024-the-publics-use-and-views-of-glp-1-drugs/
2. Aronne, L. J., Sattar, N., Horn, D. B., Bays, H. E., Wharton, S., Lin, W. Y., Ahmad, N. N., Zhang, S., Liao, R., Bunck, M. C., Jouravskaya, I., Murphy, M. A., & SURMOUNT-4 Investigators (2024). Continued Treatment With Tirzepatide for Maintenance of Weight Reduction in Adults With Obesity: The SURMOUNT-4 Randomized Clinical Trial. *JAMA,* 331(1), 38–48. https://doi.org/10.1001/jama.2023.24945
3. Rubino D, Abrahamsson N, Davies M, et al. Effect of Continued Weekly Subcutaneous Semaglutide vs Placebo on Weight Loss Maintenance in Adults with Overweight or Obesity: The STEP 4 Randomized Clinical Trial. *JAMA.* 2021;325(14):1414–1425. doi:10.1001/jama.2021.3224

Chapter 12

1. National Institute on Aging. (2020, March 24). *Higher daily step count linked with lower all-cause mortality.* [Press release]. https://www.nia.nih.gov/news/higher-daily-step-count-linked-lower-all-cause-mortality
2. A fact that has not been stated loudly enough: balance training has been shown to improve cognitive health; Rogge, A-K., Röder, B., Zech, A., & Hötting, K. (2017). Balance training improves memory and spatial cognition in healthy adults. *Scientific Reports, 7*(1), 5661; Dunsky, A. (2019). The effect of balance and coordination exercises on quality of life in older adults: A mini-review. *Frontiers in Aging Neuroscience, 11,* 318. Also a little-known fact: stretching is associated with better quality of life: Araújo, C. G. S., de Souza e Silva, C. G., Kunutsor, S. K., Franlin, B. A., Laukkanen, J. A., Myers, J., Fiatarone Singh, M. A., Franca, J. F., & Castro, C. L. B. (2024). Reduced body flexibility is associated with poor survival in middle-aged men and women: A prospective cohort study. *Scandinavian Journal of Medicine & Science in Sports, 34*(8). https://doi.org/10.1111/sms.14708

3. Blask, D. E. (2009). Melatonin, sleep disturbance, and cancer risk. *Sleep Medicine Reviews, 13*(4), 257–264. https://doi.org/10.1016/j.smrv.2008.07.007
4. Walker, M. P. (2017). *Why we sleep: Unlocking the power of sleep and dreams.* Scribner.

Chapter 13

1. Vaish, A., Grossmann, T., & Woodward, A. (2008). Not all emotions are created equal: The negativity bias in social-emotional development. *Psychological Bulletin, 134*(3), 383–403. https://doi.org/10.1037/0033-2909.134.3.383
2. National Institutes of Health. (2015, August). *Positive emotions and your health.* https://newsinhealth.nih.gov/2015/08/positive-emotions-your-health
3. Feder, S. (2020, November 13). *Religious faith can lead to positive mental benefits, writes Stanford anthropologist.* Stanford Report. https://news.stanford.edu/stories/2020/11/deep-faith-beneficial-health
4. Wickham, S. (2023). Hobbies for mental health. *Nature Medicine, 29,* 2179–2180. https://doi.org/10.1038/s41591-023-02508-z
5. Williams, M., & Penman, D. (2011). *Mindfulness: An eight-week plan for finding peace in a frantic world.* Rodale.
6. Craig, H. (2019, March 20). *What are the benefits of music therapy?* Positive Psychology. https://positivepsychology.com/music-therapy-benefits/#benefits
7. Harvard T. H. Chan School of Public Health. (2024, January 2). *Time spent in nature can boost physical and mental well-being.* (2024, January 2). https://hsph.harvard.edu/news/time-spent-in-nature-can-boost-physical-and-mental-well-being/
8. *The power of pets.* (2018, February). https://newsinhealth.nih.gov/2018/02/power-pets; Weiss, C. (2021, March 7). Mayo Clinic Q&A: How owning pets can lead to a healthier lifestyle. Mayo Clinic. https://newsnetwork.mayoclinic.org/discussion/mayo-clinic-q-and-a-how-owning-pets-can-lead-to-a-healthier-lifestyle/
9. Boyes, A. (2018, February 12). 6 benefits of an uncluttered space. *Psychology Today.* https://www.psychologytoday.com/us/blog/in-practice/201802/6-benefits-uncluttered-space
10. National Institutes of Health. (2023). *Do social ties affect our health?* https://newsinhealth.nih.gov/2023/02/do-social-ties-affect-our-health; The health benefits of socializing. (2016). *Psychology Today.* https://www.psychologytoday.com/us/articles/201606/the-health-benefits-socializing
11. Mayo Clinic Staff. (2022). *Stress management: Enhance your well-being by reducing stress.* Mayo Clinic. https://www.mayoclinic.org/healthy-lifestyle/stress-management/in-depth/stress-relief/art-20044456
12. Brownstein, M. (2025, January 8). *Kindness linked to better physical health, longevity.* Harvard T. H. Chan School of Public Health. https://hsph.harvard.edu/news/kindness-linked-to-better-physical-health-longevity/#

13. Expert Market Research. (2023). *U.S. dietary supplements market reports and forecast 2025–2034*. https://www.expertmarketresearch.com/reports/united-states-dietary-supplements-market
14. Cohen, P. A., Avula, B., Katragunta, K., Travis, J. C., & Khan, I. (2023). Presence and quantity of botanical ingredients with purported performance-enhancing properties in sports supplements. *JAMA Network Open, 6*(7), e2323879. https://doi.org/10.1001/jamanetworkopen.2023.23879

Chapter 14

1. Funk, C., Kennedy, B., & Hefferon, M. (2017, February 2). *Americans' health care behaviors and use of conventional and alternative medicine*. Pew Research Center. https://www.pewresearch.org/science/2017/02/02/americans-health-care-behaviors-and-use-of-conventional-and-alternative-medicine/
2. American Thyroid Association. (n.d.). *General information/press room*. https://www.thyroid.org/media-main/press-room/
3. Guan, N., Guariglia, A., Moore, P., Xu, F., & Al-Janabi, H. (2022). Financial stress and depression in adults: A systematic review. PLoS One, *17*(2), e0264041. https://pmc.ncbi.nlm.nih.gov/articles/PMC8863240/
4. Guthrie, B., Makubate, B., Hernandez-Santiago, V., & Dreischulte, T. (2015). The rising tide of polypharmacy and drug-drug interactions: Population database analysis 1995–2010. *BMC Medicine*, (13), 1–10.
5. KFF. (2023, June 15). *KFF survey shows complexity, red tape, denials, confusion rivals affordability as a problem for insured consumers, with some saying it caused them to go without or delay care*. https://www.kff.org/health-reform/press-release/kff-survey-shows-complexity-red-tape-denials-confusion-rivals-affordability-as-a-problem-for-insured-consumers

Chapter 16

1. Burke, L. E., Wang, J., & Sevick, M. A. (2011, January). Self-monitoring in weight loss: A systematic review of the literature. *Journal of the Academy of Nutrition and Dietetics, 111*(1), 92–102. https://doi: 10.1016/j.jada.2010.10.008; Choi, S. (2023). Personal health tracking: A paradigm shift in the self-care models in nursing. *JMIR Nursing, 6*. https://doi.org/10.2196/50991; Tarver, T. (2023, August 14). Keeping score: Why tracking progress fuels success. *Psychology Today*. https://www.psychologytoday.com/us/blog/the-healthy-journey/202308/keeping-score-why-tracking-progress-fuels-success

About the Author

DR. ALICE BURRON is a dedicated health strategist, coach, and speaker committed to guiding individuals through the complexities of health challenges with empathy and expertise. Her journey to writing this book has been driven by a higher purpose; shaped by a diverse career spanning biology, genetics, and exercise physiology; and culminating in a doctorate in healthcare education and leadership.

With over two decades of experience, Dr. Burron has earned numerous certifications—including wellness and weight loss coaching, the National Diabetes Prevention Program (DPP), Tobacco Cessation Coaching (TCC), personal training, and Zumba. Her extensive work in the healthcare system includes working in pharmacy as a junior chemist, cardiac rehabilitation as an exercise physiologist, and nearly a decade in health insurance. She also served as chair of the Wyoming Governor's Council on Physical Fitness and Sports, encouraging residents of all ages to achieve their best health through physical activity. In addition, Dr. Burron designed award-winning wellness programs for large organizations, such as the hospital in Cheyenne and the State of Wyoming's "Wyoming on Wellness" initiative. These experiences give her a unique perspective on large populations' health challenges, especially in rural areas, fueling her deep-seated desire to empower others.

This book is the culmination of her lifelong dedication to blending medical, complementary, and lifestyle approaches to health. It's not just about addressing health concerns—it's about empowering individuals to navigate their health. Dr. Burron believes that by integrating logic with the power of healing modalities, individuals can reclaim their health and become the true heroes of their health journeys.

When she's not pursuing her passion for helping others, writing, or speaking, Dr. Burron enjoys immersing herself in the wild. She thrives on the challenges of being out in rugged and raw nature, including hiking in the Wyoming wilderness and the desert and hammock camping under the stars alongside the bears—survival in the wild parallels her mission to help others navigate their health challenges with confidence and resilience.